Gluten-Free
BIBLE

Publications International, Ltd.

Recipe Development: Recipes on pages 28, 34, 42 (top), 46, 56, 66, 86, 88, 92, 104 (bottom), 110, 114 (top), 126 (top), 136, 144, 154, 168 (top), 174, 178, 194, 198, 204, 216, 228, 256, 262, 266 (top), 270, 292 and 298 (top) by Laura Walsh, RD, LDN.

Photography on pages 29, 35, 43, 47, 57, 67, 87, 89, 93, 105, 111, 115, 127, 137, 145, 155, 169, 175, 179, 195, 199, 205, 217, 229, 257, 263, 267, 271, 293 and 299 by PIL Photo Studio North.

All recipes and recipe photographs copyright © Publications International, Ltd.

Pictured on the front cover: Orange Chicken Stir-Fry Over Quinoa *(page 142)*.

Pictured on the back cover *(clockwise from top left)*: Chocolate Marble & Praline Cheesecake *(page 218)*, Rice Noodles with Broccoli and Tofu *(page 116)* and Cornmeal Pecan Muffins *(page 68)*.

Photography on pages 4, 5, 8, 9, 14, 15, 20 and 21 by Shutterstock.
Photography on page 6 by Fotofolio.
Photography on pages 7 and 23 by Jupiterimages Unlimited.
Photography on pages 7 and 11 by iStockphoto.

ISBN-13: 978-1-4508-6798-6
ISBN-10: 1-4508-6798-7

Library of Congress Control Number: 2013933143

Manufactured in China.

8 7 6 5 4 3 2 1

Microwave Cooking: Microwave ovens vary in wattage. Use the cooking times as guidelines and check for doneness before adding more time.

Note: This publication is only intended to provide general information. The information is specifically not intended to be a substitute for medical diagnosis or treatment by your physician or other health care professional. You should always consult your own physician or other health care professionals about any medical questions, diagnosis, or treatment. (Products vary among manufacturers. Please check labels carefully to confirm that the products you use are free of gluten.) **Not all recipes in this book are appropriate for all people with celiac disease, gluten intolerance, food allergies or sensitivities.**

The information obtained by you from this book should not be relied upon for any personal, nutritional, or medical decision. You should consult an appropriate professional for specific advice tailored to your specific situation. PIL makes no representations or warranties, express or implied, with respect to your use of this information.

In no event shall PIL, its affiliates or advertisers be liable for any direct, indirect, punitive, incidental, special, or consequential damages, or any damages whatsoever including, without limitation, damages for personal injury, death, damage to property, or loss of profits, arising out of or in any way connected with the use of any of the above-referenced information or otherwise arising out of the use of this book.

Publications International, Ltd.

Table of Contents

Understanding Gluten

What Is Gluten Anyway?

It's not just wheat. Gluten is a protein that is found naturally in wheat, rye and barley. Gluten gives structure to the baked goods we know and love. Without it, or something to replace it, bread and cake would be sad little puddles or piles of crumbs. When yeast, baking powder or other leavening agents produce bubbles in a dough or a batter, that air is trapped by the stretchy gluten network and the baked product rises and becomes light.

Legend has it that gluten was discovered by 7th century Buddhist monks who were trying to find something to replace the texture and savor of meat in their vegetarian diets. They found that when they submerged dough made with wheat flour in water, the starch washed away. What was left behind was a gummy mass with an almost meatlike texture—gluten. Today gluten is still used to make seitan, mock duck and other meat replacement products.

Some Techie Talk

To be technically accurate, wheat gluten is composed of two proteins—gliadin and glutenin. The proteins that make up gluten in rye and barley have different scientific names but behave much the same way since they are closely related to wheat. You will sometimes hear "corn gluten" or "rice gluten" mentioned. These proteins are very different and present no problem to those with sensitivity to wheat gluten.

Celiac Disease, Gluten Intolerance and Wheat Allergies

There are many reasons people choose to avoid gluten and many forms of gluten intolerance. Celiac disease is one of the most serious. In the 1 percent of Americans diagnosed with this autoimmune disorder, exposure to even small amounts of gluten can cause intestinal damage and result in symptoms from fatigue to anemia and bone disease. It is estimated that as many as 1 out of every 133 Americans have celiac disease.

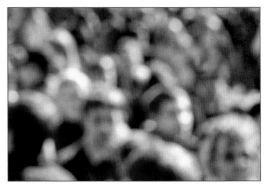

Whether you have celiac disease or another form of gluten intolerance it's good to understand the distinction. Celiac disease is a very specific condition in which exposure to gluten causes the villi, or small hairlike projections from the small intestine, to become atrophied. The purpose of these villi and the spaces between them is to let the body absorb nutrients and keep out toxins. With celiac disease, the immune system sees fragments of gluten as toxins and reacts by attacking not only the gluten but the villi themselves. An autoimmune disease, such as celiac, occurs when the body attacks itself, mistaking normal, healthy tissue for dangerous bacteria or viruses. There are more than 80 autoimmune disorders, including rheumatoid arthritis and lupus. Most, like celiac disease, are difficult to diagnose since they present a bewildering array of symptoms.

The symptoms of celiac disease and gluten sensitivity are the same. This is not surprising since they both stem from an inability to digest gluten properly. What is surprising is that there are so many different seemingly unrelated symptoms. Most people first think of gastrointestinal distress as a sign of gluten intolerance, but symptoms may also include fatigue, weight loss, weight gain, migraine headaches, anemia and sinusitis! (See the sidebar for a longer, though still not complete, list of the more than 250 possible symptoms.) Because digestion is central to providing our bodies with energy, gluten intolerance and celiac disease are multi-symptomatic. Any individual may have one or many of the possible symptoms. In fact, you can have celiac disease with no symptoms at all.

It's Complicated

Just as there are many symptoms, there are many degrees of gluten sensitivity and each person's tolerance can change over time. It is possible to develop celiac disease any time in your life for any number of reasons, including enduring a stressful period. Remember, celiac is defined as damage to the intestinal villi. You could have a genetic predisposition for the disease, which only shows up under certain circumstances. Nobody knows whether what starts out as gluten intolerance can lead to celiac disease. There are also some people who are allergic to wheat itself. A classic wheat allergy is quite different from gluten intolerance. It is likely to cause the same sorts of immediate symptoms as other food allergies—itchiness, difficulty breathing and in some cases, anaphylactic shock.

On the Other Hand, It's Simple.

Millions of Americans are going gluten-free for dozens of reasons. Some have been told that they must by their doctors. Others just feel better when they stop eating gluten. Some parents feel that a gluten-free diet improves the behavior patterns of their children,

A Not-So-Short List of Possible Symptoms

Gastrointestinal:
abdominal pain or bloating
acid reflux (GERD)
constipation
diarrhea
esophagitis
heartburn
irritable bowel syndrome
nausea
vomiting
weight loss or weight gain

Other:
acne
anemia
anxiety
canker sores
depression, irritability
dermatitis
eczema
fatigue
hair loss
inability to concentrate
infertility
irregular menstrual cycles
lactose intolerance
muscle cramps
nosebleeds
respiratory problems
sinusitis
vitamin deficiencies
  (B12, K, folate)

including those with ADHD and autism. And there are those who just think it's trendy. Truth is, if giving up gluten didn't improve so many lives, people wouldn't be willing to make the effort. There is one caveat: if you want to try gluten-free living but haven't been tested for celiac disease, you need to be tested BEFORE you start the diet. Otherwise test results will be meaningless.

Testing, Testing, One, Two, Three

Why aren't we all tested for gluten intolerance automatically? And why does it often take years to come up with a diagnosis? Part of the problem has been lack of awareness, especially in the U.S. Some European countries require children to be tested by age five and most diagnose celiac disease in a matter of months. The average time between seeing a doctor and diagnosis in the U.S. can be more than ten years, but things are improving. More doctors and medical centers are devoting some of their treatment and research to celiac disease. Unfortunately, there is no one easy, sure-fire test to detect it.

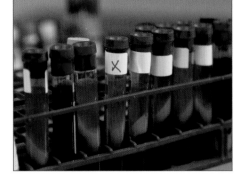

Blood samples can determine if you produce antibodies to gluten (provided you are still consuming it for several months before blood is drawn). There are five commonly used measures. None of them, unfortunately, will prove without the shadow of a doubt that you have celiac disease. If any of them is positive, your doctor may recommend a biopsy by way of endoscopy. If this determines your villi are damaged, then there is no doubt that you have celiac disease and must go on a gluten-free diet for life.

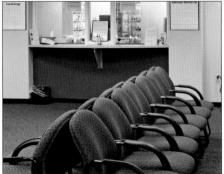

It is possible to be genetically predisposed to celiac disease, too. If you have the disease in your family, the chances are greater that you will be affected. There is also a test for genetic markers for celiac disease. If you are lacking those genes, you won't get celiac. However, not everyone who has those genes will get sick.

Your best resource is a doctor or clinic with experience in gluten intolerance and celiac disease. Just remember—if you stop eating gluten before the tests, they will be useless. On the other hand, if you feel better when you don't eat gluten, maybe test results aren't that important.

How Can Wheat Suddenly Be Bad for Us?

How could the staff of life turn into a health hazard? Is going gluten-free just the latest diet fad? It's wise to remember that the vast majority of the population can eat all the gluten they want and never have a problem. Those with gluten intolerance simply cannot and it does seem that their number is increasing.

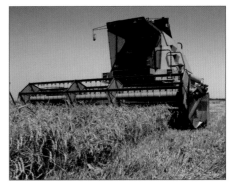

Although no one knows for sure, one factor may be that our diet today is dominated by grain, something our long-ago ancestors lived without. Wheat can feed large populations a large number of calories on relatively little land with modern agricultural methods. Of course, it also tastes good!

If you think that you don't eat much gluten because you don't eat a lot of bread, think again. Gluten is in different forms and in all sorts of processed foods. It is used as a meat substitute, a filler and to improve the texture of everything from bubble gum to ketchup. So chances are you are consuming a lot more gluten than your great grandparents. Could that be why a recent study done by the Mayo Clinic found that gluten intolerance is four times more common today than it was in the 1950s?

Living Without

Eliminating gluten from your life is not easy, nor is it a short-term proposition. There is no pill for gluten intolerance and no treatment other than changing your diet for good. On the other hand, feeling healthy and energetic for the first time in years can be a huge reward for the effort. At first glance, the list of what you must give up can seem daunting—pasta, bread, crackers, bagels, pretzels, pizza, donuts, even chicken nuggets! The good news is that there are many more foods on the gluten-free list than on the forbidden one. There are also more products, from cereals to baking mixes to pastas, which are now being formulated in gluten-free versions. These days you'll find them not just in health food stores and on websites, but also on the shelves of major supermarkets.

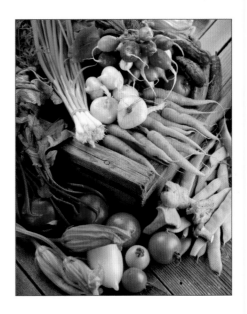

Eating gluten-free can mean eating a healthier diet—more fruits and vegetables, less processed food. You may be forced out of your old routine into doing more cooking at home and trying out new ingredients. With a bit of help from the recipes in this book, you just might find your new life is full of delicious surprises.

THE GLUTEN GUESSING GAME

It's hard enough to eliminate the obvious gluten in your life. What makes the journey tougher is that gluten hides in many places you'd never expect. Try playing our Gluten Guessing Game to test your knowledge.

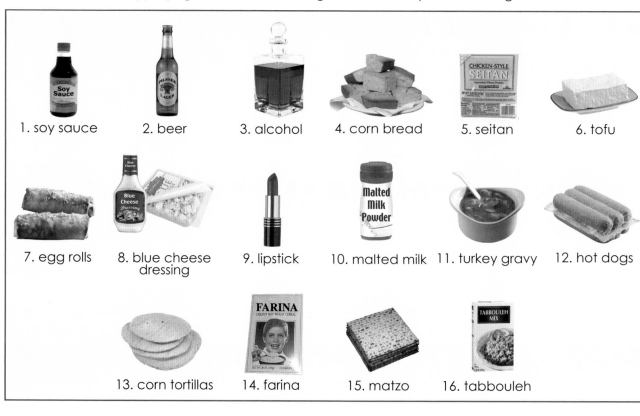

1. soy sauce   2. beer   3. alcohol   4. corn bread   5. seitan   6. tofu

7. egg rolls   8. blue cheese dressing   9. lipstick   10. malted milk   11. turkey gravy   12. hot dogs

13. corn tortillas   14. farina   15. matzo   16. tabbouleh

Answers: Numbers 2, 4, 5, 7, 10, 11, 14, 15 and 16 contain gluten. Numbers 3, 6 and 13 do NOT contain gluten. Numbers 1, 8, 9 and 12 are "maybes."

Number 1: Soy sauce is usually made with wheat; however there are some brands that are gluten-free. Tamari, which is a kind of Japanese soy sauce, is sometimes gluten-free, but read the label carefully.

Number 8: Blue cheese dressing is generally gluten-free. Blue cheese was questionable for many years since it is made with a mold that

can be derived from bread. Recent studies have shown that it is safe. Even if the starter contains wheat, the gluten remaining in the finished product is practically undetectable. Some prepared salad dressings can contain other kinds of gluten, though, so check labels.

Number 9: Lipstick and other cosmetics may contain gluten. Since lipstick is most likely to be ingested, it's wise to check the label.

Number 12: Most, but NOT all, hot dogs and other sausages are gluten-free. Once again, it's important to check the labels.

Don't Despair if You Didn't Ace the Test

You'll quickly get the hang of spotting the most obvious offenders—anything with "wheat" in its name. The most confusion arises from ingredients that are derived from gluten-containing grains. These culprits most often show up in processed foods. You never have to worry about fresh fruits, veggies, unprocessed meats or poultry.

If giving up wheat seems too difficult, remember that many of the world's great cuisines barely use wheat at all. Rice and soy are the basis for Asian cooking. Native Americans relied on what they called the "three sisters," corn, beans and squash. In fact, wheat is a relatively recent addition to our foodways. There are many delicious, nutritious grains and starches that can replace it.

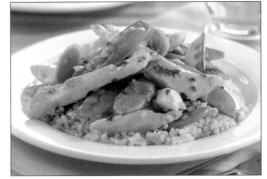
Orange Chicken Stir-Fry Over Quinoa (page142)

The best way to go gluten-free is to make the switch to a better overall diet. Start by checking out the red light/green light chart of foods on the next page.

The Never-Ending Oat Controversy

Oats have been on and off the gluten-free list for years. The main problem is that most oats are processed in facilities that also handle wheat products and are contaminated for that reason. There are brands of certified gluten-free oats available (at a premium price) that have been farmed, processed and packed in a dedicated facility. These are safe for most everyone. However, there seems to be a small subset of celiac patients who have a problem with a protein present in oats. Research is still underway.

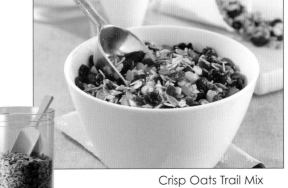
Crisp Oats Trail Mix (page 310)

No More Crying in Your Beer

Beer lovers can rejoice! Since beer is traditionally made with barley, it used to be off limits to the gluten intolerant. These days more and more small craft brewers as well as major companies are tapping into the huge market for gluten-free products. They're brewing beer made from sorghum, millet, rice and other grains. There are already at least half a dozen breweries in the U.S. alone so you should be able to fill a frosty mug to your liking.

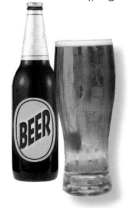

THE SHORT LIST
Sensitivities differ from person to person and ingredients differ from brand to brand. Always check the label's fine print. This is an abbreviated list of some of the most common items.

RED LIGHTS: (contain gluten)

barley	durum	kamut	rye
beer	einkorn	malt vinegar	seitan
bran	emmer	malt, malt flavoring, malt extract	semolina
brewer's yeast	graham		spelt
bulgur	gravies and sauces	matzo	tabbouleh
commercial baked goods	hydrolyzed wheat protein	orzo	wheat
couscous	imitation seafood	pizza	
		pretzels	

Yellow Lights: (may contain gluten)

artificial color*	cereal	hydrolyzed plant protein (HPP)	oats (see page 9)
baking powder	dextrins*		pasta sauce
barbecue sauce	emulsifiers	marinades	salad dressings
caramel color*	flavorings	modified food starch*	soba noodles
canned or packaged broth	frozen vegetables with sauce/seasonings	mustard	soy sauce
		nondairy creamer	

These items are gluten-free if made in the U.S. or Canada

Green Lights: (no gluten)

almond flour	corn, cornmeal	meat and poultry	sorghum flour
baking soda	corn grits	millet	soy, soy flour
beans	corn tortillas	mono and diglycerides	sweet rice flour (glutinous rice flour)
buckwheat	dairy	nuts	tapioca
carob	distilled alcohol	oils and fats	tofu
carrageenan	eggs	polenta	vegetables (fresh, canned or frozen without sauce/ seasonings)
cellophane noodles (bean thread noodles)	fruit, fresh, frozen or dried	potatoes	
	guar gum	quinoa	vinegar (except malt)
cheese	lentils	rice, rice flour	xanthan gum
chickpea flour (garbanzo flour, besan flour)	maltodextrin	rice noodles	
	masa harina	seafood	

ADVANCED LABEL READING

Spotting the gluten in foods is considerably easier now than ever before. Since 2004, the FDA's Food Allergy Labeling Law has required that any product containing wheat or derived from it must say so on the label. This means that many ingredients that used to be questionable, such as modified food starch and maltodextrin, must now show wheat as part of their name if they were made from it (for example, "wheat maltodextrin"). This law also applies to all eight of the most common allergens—eggs, fish, milk, peanuts, tree nuts, shellfish, soybeans and wheat. The only catch is that some sources of gluten, namely barley and rye, are NOT common allergens and don't have to be labeled. Also, you need to be aware that this ONLY applies to foods produced in the U.S. and Canada. Imports are a different matter.

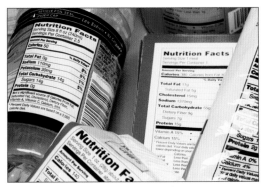

Becoming a Label Detective

Going gluten-free means you may have to start bringing a magnifying glass on your shopping trips. At the very least, you will learn a great deal about the many ingredients that go into all the processed food most of us take for granted. You may even decide that paying attention to the ingredients list is a lot more relevant than some of the marketing hype that appears on the front of the package.

The red flag you're searching for is the word "wheat." If anything in the product contains, or is made from wheat, by law it must be listed as such. Next, look for any ingredients you don't recognize. Chances are you'll find a few multisyllabic words that sound like they came from the chemistry lab. You'll need to check a list of safe and unsafe ingredients to figure those out. (You can even download such lists for your smart phone these days.

Soon enough, you'll recognize the most common ones that can be a problem (even if you never do learn how to pronounce them).

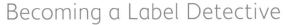

Once Is Not Enough

Product formulations change frequently. Don't assume just because you've used a brand or product in the past that it is necessarily safe or not safe forever. Don't hesitate to contact the manufacturer if you have questions about ingredients. Most companies are eager to accommodate their gluten-free customers and many list the information on their websites. Call the customer service help line or visit the website. You'll get the information and maybe even a few coupons for your trouble.

Does a Gluten-Free Label Mean 100% Gluten-Free?

The short answer is not exactly. Experts agree that food can contain a very small amount of gluten and still be tolerated by even those who are sensitive. The trouble is, not everyone agrees on exactly what that tiny amount should be.

The FDA is doing studies and soliciting consumer input on a definition for gluten-free that will eventually govern what appears on labels. For international trade, standards have been set at less than 20 parts per million so that is often the assumed threshold. Meanwhile, there is a private, not-for-profit certification program in place that tests products to see if they contain less than 10 parts per million of gluten. Those that do are allowed to display a "Certified Gluten-Free" logo. Remember, most food is naturally gluten-free. There's no need to look for GF labels on dairy products or a can of beans!

GLUTEN-FREE NUTRITION

Is Gluten-Free Healthier?

If you are suffering from celiac disease or gluten intolerance it certainly is! One of the many devastating effects can be the inability of damaged intestines to derive the nutrients your body needs. However, there are steps you should take to ensure you get proper nutrition on a gluten-free diet. Begin by talking to your doctor. Chances are, he or she can suggest a Registered Dietitian you can consult who specializes in gluten-free eating.

The Saga of Soy Sauce

Traditional Chinese soy sauce is brewed from soybeans and wheat, so it's off limits. There are some brands that skip the brewing process and use soy concentrate and caramel coloring instead. The good news is that these GF soy sauces are cheaper, but they do lack flavor and complexity.

Tamari is a particular kind of Japanese soy sauce. Some tamari does contain wheat, however, there is a major brand that offers a certified gluten-free, wheat-free tamari. Another option is to substitute a liquid amino concentrate available at health food stores. Bottom line is always check the label!

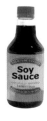

Top 10 Tips for Healthier GF Eating

1. Remember that "gluten-free" on the label doesn't always mean it's healthy.

2. Don't gorge on GF brownies and cookies, even when you find some that are delicious.

3. Don't overdo starches like rice, potatoes and corn.

4. Eat gluten-free whole grains—brown rice, whole grain cornmeal, quinoa, etc.

5. In flour mixes, look for nutritious amaranth, millet, buckwheat, montina, sorghum or teff flour.

6. Get enough fiber from whole fruits, beans, lentils and chickpeas.

7. Go global. Asian, South American, Mediterranean and Indian cuisines offer many nutritious and gluten-free dishes and ingredients.

8. Stock your kitchen and your pantry with quality ingredients and cooking equipment.

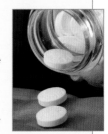

9. Get your B vitamins. In your old life, enriched white flour provided some of them. Ask your doctor if you should take a supplement.

10. Protein is important and it's gluten-free! Enjoy lean meats, seafood and tofu.

Gluten-Free Is Not Low-Calorie, Fat-Free or Low-Carb

It is most certainly not a weight-loss regimen. If you simply replace the old white bread, cakes and cookies with gluten-free versions of the same thing, you might be worse off! Most ordinary white flour is fortified to make up for the nutrients lost during processing. Some processed gluten-free flours are nutritionally empty starches. For instance, white rice flour has considerably fewer B vitamins, iron and folate than enriched white flour. It does have more refined carbohydrate, though—not a good trade-off!

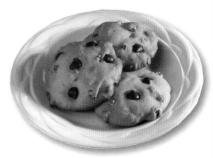

On the other hand, going gluten-free can be the start of a healthier diet. You will certainly be paying more attention to the food you eat, which is a huge step in the right direction. Instead of trying to replicate your old diet, start fresh—eat more fresh fruits, vegetables, lean meat and low-fat dairy. If that sounds familiar, it is. It's the basic dietary advice given to everyone, gluten-free or not. Think of your GF lifestyle as an opportunity to try new things, not a life sentence that will deprive you of foods you used to love.

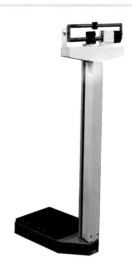

Weighing In on Gluten-Free

Some people gain weight after going gluten-free, some lose. Many newly diagnosed celiac patients are sickly and undernourished because of their disease. Once their bodies begin healing, they regain weight and strength. As gluten-free eating has become mainstream, some people try it hoping to lose weight. As with most popular diets, this is only successful if you are eating fewer calories and replacing empty ones with food that is more nutritious.

THE GLUTEN-FREE KITCHEN

How to Start Your New Life

Eating gluten-free means the days of ordering a pizza or picking up a bucket of fried chicken for dinner at the last minute are over. Don't despair! You are about to encounter a whole new world of flavors and good things to eat. GF cooking isn't difficult—it's just different. The biggest change may be that you need to cook more and use processed foods less.

For those recently diagnosed with celiac disease, setting up the kitchen to avoid cross contamination is an important first step. If you live alone, purge your place of breads, pastas, flours and other no-no's. If you are living with gluten-eating others, you'll need to stake out a GF zone of your own. The biggest culprit in cross-contamination is the common crumb. Crumbs from regular bread find their way onto work surfaces, into condiment jars and toasters. You will have to clearly mark GF items and make sure everyone understands they are hands-off. Dishes and pots and pans can be shared, because they can be washed between uses. If you will be toasting GF and regular bread, you may want to invest in a second toaster to make your life easier.

Wheat-Free Is Not Gluten-Free

When you find a product marked "gluten-free" you can be sure you're in safe territory. Wheat-free, however, is no guarantee. The product could contain gluten from barley, rye, oats or something derived from them. Remember, wheat is considered an allergen and must be labeled. The others are not.

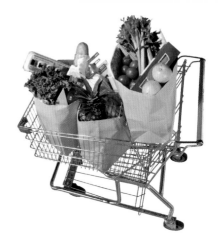

Supermarket Savvy

Before you rush off to buy a cupboard full of specialty products, remember that most basic ingredients are naturally gluten-free. You can pick up any sort of fresh produce, meat or fish without worrying. However, macaroni and cheese from a box and fish sticks are no longer on your list. This doesn't mean you can't have your favorite foods anymore. It just means you will be making some adjustments.

Impulse shopping isn't a great option either. Most supermarkets stock huge displays with brightly colored boxes of highly processed, gluten-filled items. It may also amaze you how many aisles you can skip when you no longer wander aimlessly amidst the latest bread, cracker and snack items.

Of course, you will want to stock up on certain things so that you're prepared to eat well on your new diet. Five years ago a health food store was the only place to buy specialty flours and mixes. Fortunately, today most supermarkets offer just about everything you need. There are also many reliable online sources that are worth checking out.

THE GLUTEN-FREE PANTRY

Cooking gluten-free is easier if you keep these staples on hand.

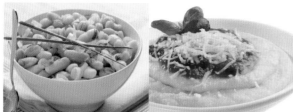
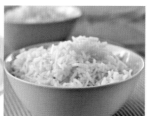

- ☐ beans and lentils
- ☐ chickpea flour
- ☐ corn grits
- ☐ corn tortillas and taco shells
- ☐ cornmeal and cornstarch
- ☐ GF cereal (corn and/or rice)
- ☐ GF flour blends (page 19)
- ☐ GF mixes for your favorite brownies, cookies or muffins
- ☐ GF pasta in various shapes
- ☐ GF soy sauce
- ☐ polenta
- ☐ quinoa
- ☐ rice (arborio, basmati)
- ☐ rice flour (brown, white and sweet)
- ☐ rice noodles
- ☐ tapioca flour
- ☐ wild rice
- ☐ xanthan gum

What Is Xanthan Gum Anyway?

It sounds mysterious, doesn't it? Xanthan gum is a chain of polysaccharides (for the nonchemists that's a chain of sugars) made by fermenting a carbohydrate (often corn sugar). Xanthan gum was approved for use as a food additive in 1968 and is used as a thickener and stabilizer in salad dressings, ice cream, low-fat dairy products and, of course, gluten-free baked goods.

In the Thick of It

From apple pie to white sauce, wheat flour is often used to thicken things. That's partly because it's cheap and readily available. There are plenty of gluten-free substitutes that offer real advantages. Tapioca flour, arrowroot and sweet rice flour (mochiko) thicken sauces and pie fillings beautifully. They also tolerate freezing and thawing better than those thickened with flour or cornstarch.

Keeping Expenses Under Control

The first time you see the price on a package of xanthan gum or gluten-free pretzels you may feel faint. Many people complain about the cost of going gluten-free, but there are ways to control spending. The biggest budget busters tend to be specialty goods, such as gluten-free cookies, cakes and snacks. It's comforting to see familiar goodies that are made just for you, and tempting to overindulge, but plenty of your old favorites are naturally gluten-free, including most potato chips, corn chips and candy.

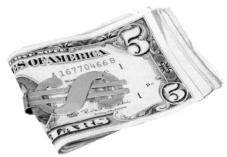

Because gluten-free is a hot topic, there are also some products that have always been gluten-free now sporting a gluten-free label and costing more. Don't pay extra for vanilla extract that's labeled gluten-free when all vanilla is!

Once you figure out which gluten-free ingredients you will need in quantity—for example flours for blends—buy in bulk. You will find many grains available in the bulk bins at the supermarket. It pays to search out online sources, as well. You can purchase millet or almond flour for a lot less per pound in a five-pound bag. If you don't have a need or the storage space for big quantities, share a shipment with gluten-free friends.

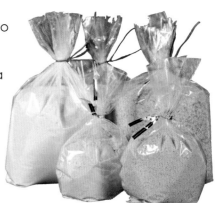

Many cultures and millions of people around the world thrive on diets with little or no gluten. In fact, ethnic markets are often great sources for well-priced gluten-free foods. Rice flour will cost less at an Asian grocer since it is in much greater demand. The same holds true for cornmeal at a Latin American market or polenta at an Italian deli. Instead of only trying to find gluten-free versions of the same old foods, use the diet as an opportunity to explore new ones.

Simple Trade-Offs

Instead of...	Try...
breakfast oatmeal	Breakfast Quinoa (page 42)
fried fish fillets	Fish and "Chips" (page 208)
chicken nuggets	Extra Crunchy Chicken Tenders (page 280)
lasagna	Creamy Layered Vegetable Bake (page 154)
egg rolls	Vietnamese Summer Rolls (page 102)
Mexican carry-out	Beef & Bean Enchiladas (page 140)
apple pie	Best Ever Apple Crisp (page 216)

BAKING GLUTEN-FREE AND EASY

There's no need to give away your old cookbooks and recipe cards. Many recipes don't have any problematic ingredients or can easily be converted. When small quantities of flour are needed—for example, to bread chicken or fish—you can substitute any gluten-free flour for regular flour. Stock up on ready-made GF pastas and your old Italian favorites are as easy as ever.

Baked goods, especially breads, are a whole lot trickier. While it is certainly possible to buy premade GF cookies, cakes and breads, they are expensive and can't compete with homemade treats. Fortunately, it is possible to turn out luscious gluten-free brownies, cakes, pies and even bread with the recipes in this book and a bit of practice. In fact, warm GF bread from your oven is probably tastier and better for you than most supermarket wheat breads!

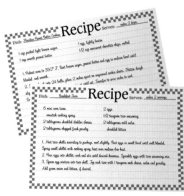

Flour Power

You won't be surprised to learn that the trick to making GF baked goods is finding a way to replace the power of gluten. In order to replicate the structure and texture it provides, you'll need to combine different nonwheat flours and add xanthan gum. While you can buy premade GF all-purpose flour blends as well as mixes for anything from pancakes to chocolate cake, it's helpful to know a little about the actual flours in them. It seems there are new choices available every day—hemp flour and pea flour are two of the latest.

Here are descriptions of some of the more common ones.

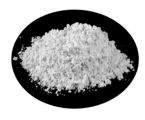

Almond Flour has a sweet, nutty flavor that complements cookies and cakes. You can make your own almond flour by pulverizing blanched nuts in a food processor. It is very easy to end up with almond butter, though, so beware! Almond flour is low in carbohydrates and high in protein. It is a classic ingredient in Passover cooking.

Chickpea Flour is also called garbanzo flour or besan flour. This hearty flour is high in protein, fiber and calcium. You'll find it in many Indian, Italian and Mediterranean recipes and it is an excellent addition to flour blends.

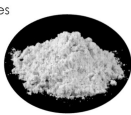

Coconut Flour is low in carbohydrates and high in fiber. It has a subtle coconut fragrance and flavor. Coconut flour absorbs a lot of liquid and can easily become dense. Recipes usually call for a small amount of coconut flour and more eggs than usual.

Corn Flour is the finely ground form of cornmeal. Masa harina, which is milled from hominy (corn treated with slaked lime) is a special kind of corn flour used to make tortillas and in other Mexican recipes. There is also a special corn flour which is precooked and labeled masarepa or masa al instante.

Cornmeal comes in a variety of grinds and colors, from fine to coarse, and in white, yellow and even blue! It's perfect for corn muffins, polenta and breading among other things. Cornmeal is nutritious and has a nutty, sweet flavor. Using too coarse a grind can produce gritty baked goods.

Cornstarch has probably always been in your pantry. A fine white powder, cornstarch is highly refined and used as a thickener and a bland ingredient that lightens many GF flour blends.

Millet Flour is made from a cereal grain that is used in African and Indian cuisine. (Whole millet is also used as bird food!) It is mild in flavor and easy to digest. Millet's mild flavor, plus a high fiber and protein content make it work well in blends for yeast breads.

Rice Flour (white or brown) is the most commonly used gluten-free flour and a good one-to-one substitute in recipes that only call for a tablespoon or two of regular flour. Like the rice it is made from, brown rice flour is whole grain, so it is nutritionally better, but makes things heavier.
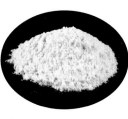

Rice Flour, Sweet can be confusing, since it's sometimes called glutinous rice flour! It does not contain gluten, but is made from short grain "sticky" rice. The Japanese term for this flour is mochiko since it is used in making mochi (rice cakes). It is an excellent thickener but has little nutritional value.

Sorghum Flour is sometimes called milo or jowar flour, and is a relatively new and very welcome addition to the gluten-free pantry. It is nutritious and high in protein so it works well in flour blends for breads. Many find the flavor similar to regular wheat flour.
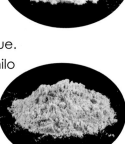

Soy Flour is ground from roasted soybeans. Choose defatted soy flour. Regular is extremely perishable and prone to rancidity. Soy flour is high in protein, but it has a distinctive "beany" flavor many people don't like.

Tapioca Flour is often labeled tapioca starch. It comes from the root of the cassava (manioc) plant. You are probably more familiar with tapioca pearls used to make pudding, which come from the same root but are processed differently. Tapioca flour gives a bit of chewiness to GF baked goods and is also an excellent thickener.

FLOUR BLENDS AND FRIENDS

Why can't there be a single one-for-one substitute for wheat flour? Unfortunately wheat flour performs many different functions and is made up of both protein (the gluten) and starches. It helps make pie crusts flaky, cookies chewy and breads crusty. There is no one GF flour that can recreate all those benefits, but that's no reason to give up baking. With two basic flour blends in your refrigerator you can turn out yummy cakes, cookies and even yeast breads. Here are the blends used for many of the recipes in this book.

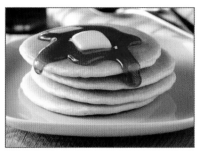

Buttermilk Pancakes
(page 26)

GLUTEN-FREE ALL-PURPOSE FLOUR BLEND

(This blend is for all baked goods not made with yeast.)

1 cup white rice flour
1 cup sorghum flour
1 cup tapioca flour
1 cup cornstarch
1 cup almond flour or coconut flour

Combine all ingredients in a large bowl. Whisk to make sure the flours are evenly distributed. The recipe can be doubled or tripled. Store in an airtight container in the refrigerator.

GLUTEN-FREE FLOUR BLEND FOR BREADS

(This blend is for recipes that call for yeast.)

1 cup brown rice flour
1 cup sorghum flour
¾ cup millet flour*
1 cup tapioca flour
1 cup cornstarch
⅓ cup instant mashed potato flakes (unflavored)

If millet flour is not available, chickpea flour may be substituted.

Combine all ingredients in a large bowl. Whisk to make sure flours are evenly distributed. The recipe can be doubled or tripled. Store in an airtight container in the refrigerator.

Fiber Factoids

Most of us don't get enough fiber in our diets. Here's a list of some common GF flours and their fiber content, from high to low.

FLOUR	FIBER PER 1 CUP
Chickpea flour	20.9 grams
Almond flour	14.7 grams
Millet flour	10.3 grams
Brown rice flour	7.3 grams
White rice flour	3.8 grams
Cornstarch	1.2 grams
Tapioca	0 grams

Blending the Rules

While gluten-free flour blends may seem mysterious at first, they do follow certain rules. Basic all-purpose flour blends usually start with two parts of grain flour (rice, sorghum or millet), two parts of starch (cornstarch or tapioca flour) and one part of protein flour (a bean or nut). There are many other considerations like flavor and nutrition. While a blend made of white rice flour and cornstarch might work, it wouldn't contain much in the way of fiber, protein or vitamins. You can, of course, purchase ready-made blends at the supermarket or on the Internet, but homemade is certainly cheaper and also fresher and better tasting.

Storing and Using GF Flour Blends

Most gluten-free flour blends should be stored in the refrigerator or freezer since they contain perishable whole grain or nut flours. Invest in canisters or use clearly marked resealable freezer bags. Bring flours to room temperature before using and remember to rewhisk or shake them so that they are completely combined.

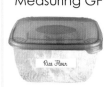

Measuring GF blends is no different than measuring wheat flour, but it is even more important to be accurate. Never pack flour into a measuring cup. Don't dip the measuring cup into the flour, either, since that can compact it. Fluff the flour and spoon it into the cup. Level off the top with the back of a knife.

BAKING TIPS AND TRICKS

Gluten-free baking isn't harder, it's just different. The good/bad news is that you'll probably be doing more baking now that you're gluten-free. That's good because you won't be eating all of the questionable ingredients in most packaged breads and cookies. The bad news is that you'll have to find the time. There is a bit of a learning curve to gluten-free baking, so don't be discouraged by a failure. Remember, you probably failed at traditional baking a few times, too! Many products that may not look as beautiful as you would like will still taste very good. You can also turn a total failure into gluten-free crumbs to be used another time.

Mixing Mastery

Gather all the flours you'll need to make a blend and get out your largest bowl.

Many flours, especially the starchy ones, look alike. Pay close attention and check off each ingredient as you go. Blend the flours thoroughly with a whisk.

Don't Gum Things Up!

If you use a store-bought flour blend, be sure to check the ingredients. Some contain xanthan or guar gum already. You do not want to double the amount of gum in a recipe. The recipes in this book assume that you are using a blend WITHOUT xanthan or guar gum.

Think Different

Many batters and doughs look drastically different from their gluten-containing counterparts. They tend to be wetter and stickier. Bread dough is more like a thick, stretchy batter. You can celebrate the fact that you'll never need to knead GF bread dough. That's a good thing, since it's so sticky you'd never be able to! You will need to learn to shape sticky dough by using damp hands or a well-oiled spoon or spatula. Parchment paper can be a real help for lining pans and transporting soft doughs.

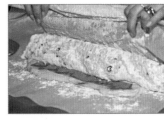

You will be using xanthan gum to provide elasticity and hold doughs together. It's important to measure it very carefully. Too much and your baked goods will shrink after baking and you may find a dense, gummy layer of dough near the bottom of the pan.

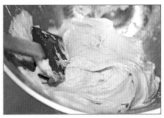

Smarty Pans

Pans are a critical part of the recipe. Black or dark metal pans can be a problem because they absorb heat more quickly. The recipes in this book were tested in pans and on baking sheets with light, shiny surfaces. If you must use dark pans, try lining them with foil, watch carefully and lower oven temperatures or cooking times, if necessary. Disposable aluminum pans work surprisingly well for many recipes.

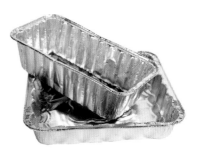

Pan size can be the difference between a perfect cake or loaf and a flop—literally! The same batter intended for a 9×5-inch loaf pan can puff up over the top of an 8×4-inch pan and then collapse. Measure pan size across the top from inside edge to inside edge.

Temperamental Temperatures

Oven temperatures are also important. If you don't have an oven thermometer, you may want to get one. Home ovens are frequently off by as much as 50 degrees. While you're at it, pick up an inexpensive instant-read thermometer, too. It's a big help in knowing when bread is done (190° to 200°F). Gluten-free goods tend to brown more quickly. They can look done on the outside when they're still gooey in the center so be ready to cover things with a sheet of foil to prevent burning.

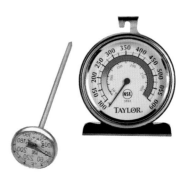

Trouble-Shooting

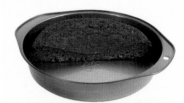

Cake left in a hot pan too long can collapse.

Problem: The cake looked gorgeous when it came out of the oven, but it fell in the center and got mushy.

Solution: Gluten-free baked goods need to be removed from pans quickly or the residual steam can cause them to collapse. Remove them from the pan to a wire rack 5 minutes after they come out of the oven.

Problem: The muffins collapsed over the top of the pan.

Solution: There may have been too much liquid in the batter. Gluten-free flours absorb less liquid than wheat flour.

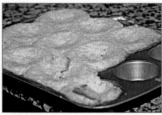

Too much liquid can make muffins collapse.

Problem: The bread was dry and hard the next morning.

Solution: GF breads stale very quickly. Always keep them well wrapped once they're cool and store in the refrigerator or freezer.

Problem: The bread was burned outside but raw in the middle.

Solution: Try lowering the oven temperature by 25 degrees. Don't bake GF breads in black, glass or nonstick-coated pans. If the outside is browning too fast, cover the bread with foil.

Problem: The cookies crumbled!

Solution: Did you remember the xanthan gum? Without it GF flours lack the elasticity to hold regular baked goods together

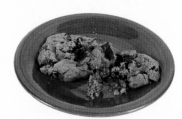

Without xanthan gum, baked goods crumble.

Problem: The bread was tough.

Solution: Beating dough for several minutes can lighten it by beating in air. Be sure to beat for the time called for in the recipe. Using a heavy duty stand mixer may help as well. You may also need to reduce the amount of flour.

Problem: The bread looked gorgeous when it came out of the oven, but then it leaned over and folded.

Solution: Don't let your GF bread rise higher than the top of the pan and don't use too small a pan.

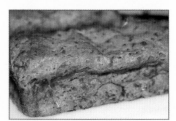

Don't let bread rise higher than the top of the pan, or it will slump.

HAPPY, HEALTHY GLUTEN-FREE KIDS

How do you explain to your child that he or she can't have a piece of Johnny's birthday cake or that those chocolate chip cookies that smell so good are off limits? It sounds impossible. Most parents would much rather make sacrifices themselves than ask their children to make them. Kids are, fortunately, considerably more resilient than we think and a gluten-free lifestyle has many positive benefits even from a pint-size perspective. Chances are this change in diet is going to be a lot harder on you than on your child.

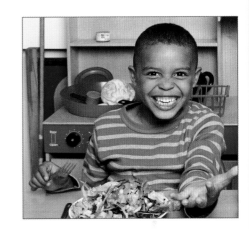

You Are Not Alone

See your child's doctor and make sure the right tests are done for celiac disease, gluten-intolerance and any other food sensitivities. Celiac does run in families, so if you or a close relative has the disease, it's more likely that others do as well. Seek out local support groups or search online for information and assistance in raising your gluten-free child.

Make it Positive

Children pick up on adult attitudes and emotions (at least until they are teenagers!). They are also quite adept at knowing when you are trying to convince them of something you don't believe. Just try to make your kid eat broccoli if you loathe it yourself! You need to appreciate the benefits of living gluten-free first. The major plus is better health now and for the future.

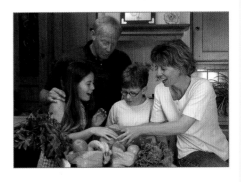

Many symptoms will improve almost immediately. Help your child understand that the reason his tummyaches went away is that he is now gluten-free. Instead of focusing on what is forbidden, emphasize the delicious gluten-free good things on the menu. Show them some of the photos of the yummy treats you'll be making from Chapter 10, "Kiddie Creations." They may even volunteer to help you bake.

Eight Tips to Ease the Way

1. Give Them Control. The more your child understands the GF diet and the reasons for it, the better. Sooner or later he will have to make decisions when you're not around.

2. Spread the Word. Make baby-sitters, friends' parents, relatives and school officials aware that your child is on the GF diet and that it is extremely important he sticks to it.

3. Explain How to Explain. It can be something simple, like "I'm allergic to gluten." The more a child feels comfortable talking about dietary restrictions, the safer he is.

4. Find Alternatives. You will not be able to replace brownies with broccoli. Instead bake Classic Brownies (page 234) or offer another gluten-free treat.

5. Party Plan. If your son or daughter is invited to a birthday party or sleepover, send along a gluten-free replacement for whatever is being served. Explain the situation to the parent in charge and let them know what you're sending.

6. School Daze. Ask the teacher to keep a stash of gluten-free goodies on hand so when there's a celebration involving food, he won't feel left out.

7. Use Mistakes. We all make them. If your child accidentally (or on purpose) eats gluten, don't berate him. If eating it made him feel lousy, though, point it out.

8. Don't Make it a Big Deal. It is a big deal for you, but a kid's world is filled with friends, pets, bikes, superheroes and recess. They are probably not obsessing about food like you are, and that's good.

DAIRY-FREE AND GLUTEN-FREE: THE GFCF DIET

Many families are choosing a gluten-free casein-free (GFCF) diet for children with symptoms of ADD/ADHD or autism. While there is no scientific evidence that eliminating gluten and casein helps these conditions, there are many anecdotal accounts of improvements in symptoms. Why would this be so? One theory is that some children are not able to completely digest the protein in milk (casein) and wheat (gluten) and that these leftover proteins form peptides in the blood that act like opiates in the body, influencing behavior. Research in the U.S. and Europe has found peptides in the urine of a significant number of children with autism.

Studies are currently underway to see if the GFCF diet really can be proven effective. Always consult your doctor before changing your child's diet. Tests can determine sensitivities to gluten and casein and whether there are peptides present. You should also get professional dietary advice to ensure your child will be getting the nutrition he or she needs.

What Is Casein?

Casein is the primary protein in milk. (Lactose is milk sugar. It is possible to be lactose intolerant but able to handle casein, though often when one is problematic they both are.) What complicates a GFCF diet is the fact that casein is used as a binding agent in many processed foods and goes by many different chemical names.

Cooking Minus the Moo

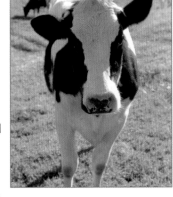

Clearly milk, cheese and butter are off the ingredient list, but did you know that most margarine contains dairy in the form of whey or casein? So do many soy cheeses. Fortunately, U.S. food manufacturers are now required to list the simple word "milk" as part of the ingredient list or in boldface type at the end of the list, even if the actual ingredient goes by an obscure chemical name. The recent popularity of the vegan diet is a boon for dairy-free shoppers, too. Since vegans consume no animal products, you can assume products labeled vegan are dairy-free. The kosher designation "pareve" is another handy indicator that the product contains no milk.

Nondairy is NOT Always Dairy-Free

Many products labeled nondairy contain whey, casein or other milk-derived ingredients. According to the FDA, nondairy products can contain 0.5 percent or less of milk products by weight. Nondairy creamers and nondairy whipped toppings usually contain dairy in some form.

Dairy Doubles

The good news is that there are more and better dairy replacement products available all the time. In addition to soymilk, you can purchase almond milk, rice milk, oat milk and even hemp milk. For most recipes, including those in this book, dairy-free milk may be substituted one-for-one for cow's milk. You may want to choose one kind of milk for drinking and another for cooking. Vanilla soymilk is delicious on its own but would be quite odd in mashed potatoes!

To replace butter in most baking recipes, choose a stick form of dairy-free margarine. Nondairy spreads sold in tubs will not always work well in baking recipes because of the softer consistency.

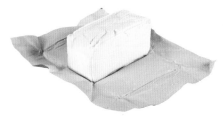

Cheese is one of the toughest things to replace. Some nondairy cheeses taste nothing like the real thing and many of them melt poorly or not at all, but there are more and better choices all the time. For bland cheeses, like ricotta or cottage cheese, crumbled tofu is often a good stand in.

All of the recipes in Chapter 11, "Allergy-Free Fare," are dairy-free as well as gluten-free. Some are also free of eggs, peanuts and/or soy. With a bit of planning and The Gluten-Free Bible, GFCF meals can be easy, nutritious and delicious.

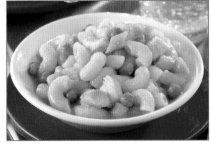

Allergy-Free Mac & Cheez
(page 304)

Breakfast Bliss

BUTTERMILK PANCAKES

Makes 16 pancakes (about 4 servings)

    2 cups Gluten-Free All-Purpose Flour Blend (page 19)*
 1½ tablespoons sugar
    1 teaspoon baking powder
    1 teaspoon baking soda
  ½ teaspoon salt
 2¼ cups low-fat buttermilk
    2 eggs
    2 tablespoons butter, melted and cooled
       Vegetable oil
       Butter and/or maple syrup

Or use any all-purpose gluten-free flour blend that does not contain xanthan gum.

1. Combine flour blend, sugar, baking powder, baking soda and salt in large bowl. Whisk buttermilk, eggs and 2 tablespoons butter in small bowl. Gradually whisk buttermilk mixture into flour mixture until smooth.

2. Heat oil on griddle or in large nonstick skillet over medium heat. Pour ¼ cupfuls of batter 2 inches apart onto griddle. Cook 2 minutes or until lightly browned and edges begin to bubble. Turn over; cook 2 minutes or until lightly browned. Repeat with remaining batter. Serve with additional butter and/or maple syrup.

Note: If you do not plan on serving the pancakes right away, keep them warm in a 200°F oven.

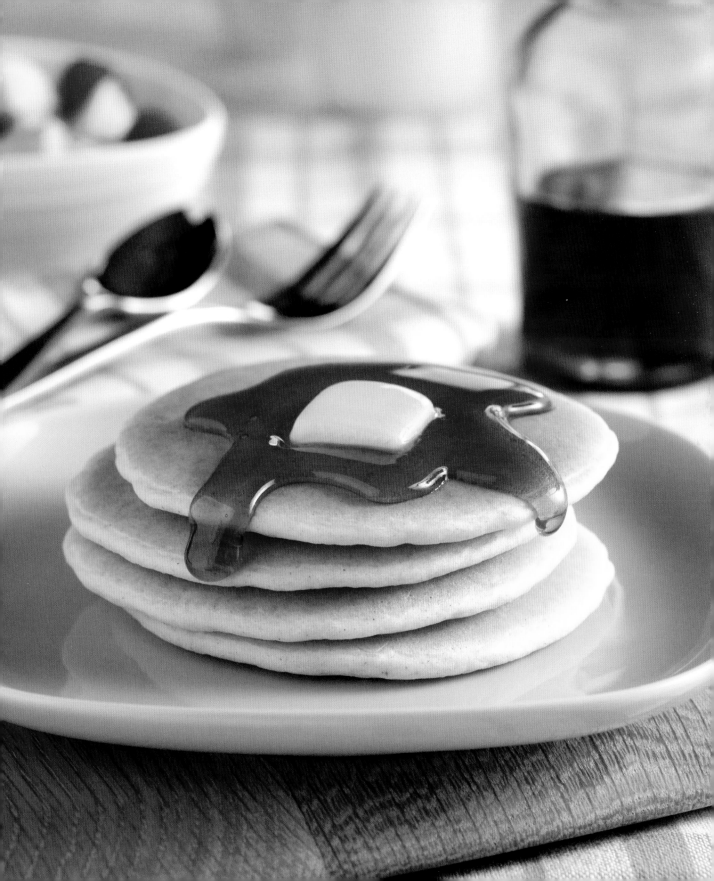

SPINACH, ARTICHOKE AND ASIAGO QUICHE

Makes 6 servings

Gluten-Free Pie Crust (recipe follows)
1½ cups half-and-half
3 eggs
1¼ cups shredded Asiago cheese, divided
¼ teaspoon salt
¼ teaspoon black pepper
¼ teaspoon ground nutmeg
2 teaspoons Dijon mustard
1 package (10 ounces) frozen chopped spinach, thawed and squeezed dry
1 cup water-packed quartered artichokes, drained, squeezed dry and chopped

1. Prepare Gluten-Free Pie Crust.

2. Preheat oven to 375°F. Lightly grease 9-inch pie pan. Place pie crust in prepared pan. Flute edge as desired. Bake 20 minutes.

3. Meanwhile, whisk half-and-half and eggs in medium bowl until well blended. Stir in ¾ cup cheese, salt, pepper and nutmeg.

4. *Reduce oven temperature to 350°F.* Spread mustard over prepared crust. Layer evenly with spinach and artichokes, pressing down lightly into crust. Pour egg mixture evenly over vegetables. Top evenly with remaining ½ cup cheese.

5. Bake 40 minutes or until knife inserted into center comes out clean. Let stand 10 minutes before serving.

Tip: If edges are browning too quickly in oven, cover with a strip of aluminum foil.

GLUTEN-FREE PIE CRUST

Makes 1 (9- to 10-inch pie crust)

1 cup Gluten-Free All-Purpose Flour Blend (page 19),* plus additional for work surface
2 tablespoons sweet rice flour (mochiko)
1½ teaspoons sugar
½ teaspoon xanthan gum
¼ teaspoon salt

continued on page 30

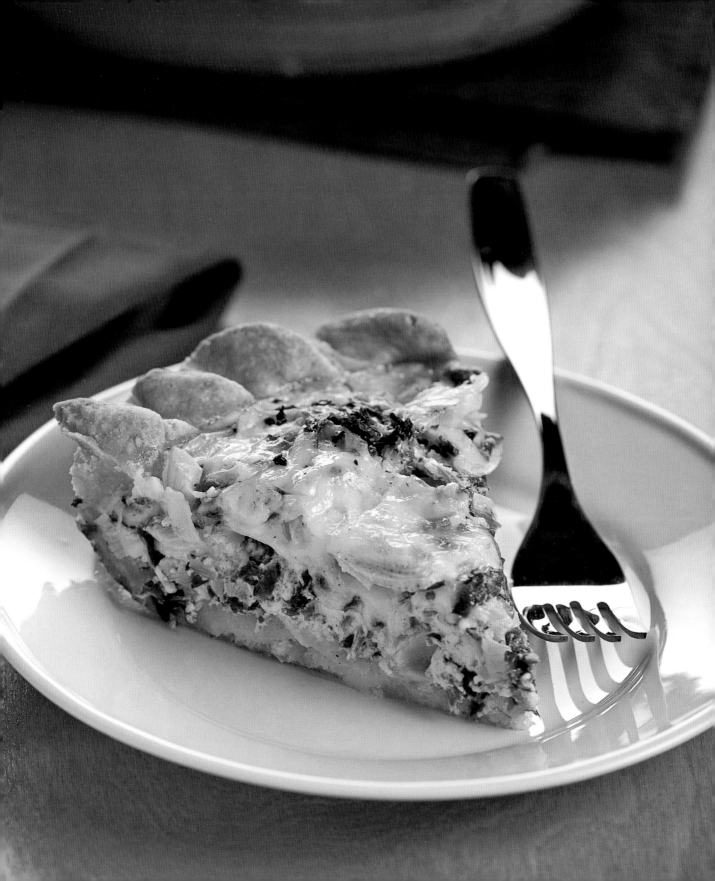

Spinach, Artichoke and Asiago Quiche, continued

> **6 tablespoons (¾ stick) cold butter, cubed**
> **1 egg**
> **2 teaspoons cider vinegar**

*Or use any all-purpose gluten-free flour blend that does not contain xanthan gum.

1. Combine 1 cup flour blend, sweet rice flour, sugar, xanthan gum and salt in medium bowl; mix well. Cut in butter with pastry blender or two knives until coarse crumbs form.

2. Make well in center of mixture. Add egg and vinegar and stir just until dough forms. Shape dough into flat disc. Wrap in plastic wrap and refrigerate at least 45 minutes or until very cold.

3. Roll out dough on floured surface into circle slightly larger than pie plate. (If dough becomes sticky, return to refrigerator until cold.) Wrap in plastic wrap and refrigerate until ready to use.

BANANA SPLIT BREAKFAST BOWL

Makes 4 servings

> **2½ tablespoons sliced almonds**
> **2½ tablespoons chopped walnuts**
> **3 cups vanilla nonfat yogurt**
> **1⅓ cups sliced strawberries (about 12 medium)**
> **2 bananas, sliced**
> **½ cup drained pineapple tidbits**

1. Spread almonds and walnuts in single layer in small heavy skillet. Cook and stir over medium heat 2 minutes or until lightly browned. Immediately remove from skillet; cool completely

2. Spoon yogurt into serving bowl. Layer with strawberries, bananas and pineapple. Sprinkle with toasted almonds and walnuts.

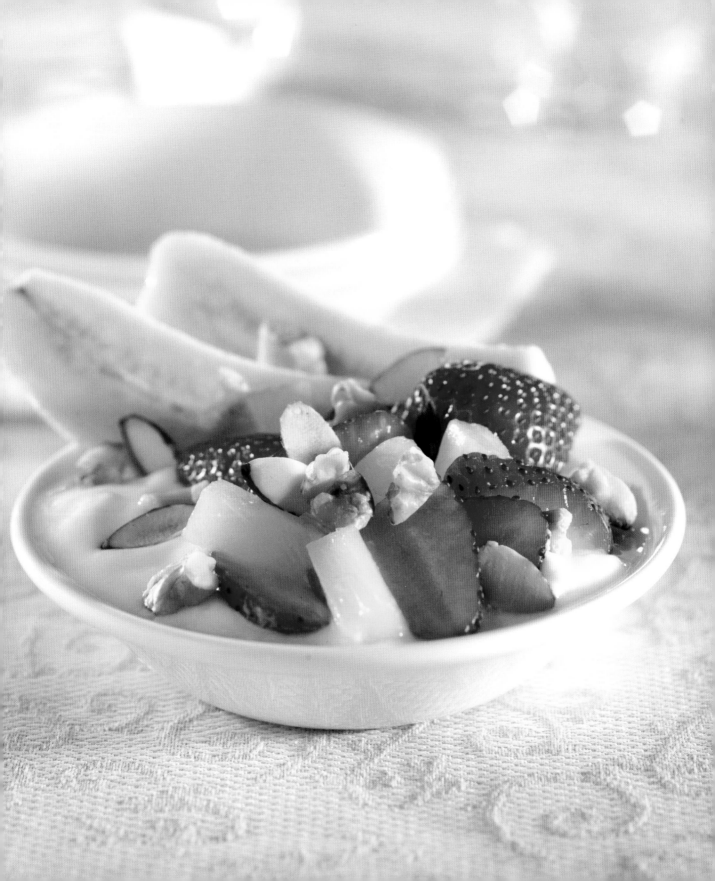

SWEET POTATO AND TURKEY SAUSAGE HASH

Makes 2 servings

    1 mild or hot turkey Italian sausage link (about 4 ounces)
    1 small red onion, finely chopped
    1 small red bell pepper, finely chopped
    1 small sweet potato, peeled and cut into ½-inch cubes
    ¼ teaspoon salt
    ¼ teaspoon black pepper
    ⅛ teaspoon cumin
    ⅛ teaspoon chipotle chili powder

1. Remove sausage from casings; discard. Shape sausage into ½-inch balls. Spray large nonstick skillet with nonstick cooking spray; heat over medium heat. Add sausage; cook and stir 3 to 5 minutes or until browned. Remove from skillet; set aside.

2. Spray same skillet with cooking spray. Add onion, bell pepper, sweet potato, salt, black pepper, cumin and chili powder; cook and stir 5 to 8 minutes or until sweet potato is tender.

3. Stir in sausage; cook without stirring 5 minutes or until hash is lightly browned.

BREAKFAST RICE PUDDING

Makes 4 servings

    2 cups vanilla soymilk, divided
    ¾ cup uncooked quick-cooking brown rice*
    ⅓ cup packed brown sugar
    ½ teaspoon ground cinnamon
    ½ teaspoon salt
    ¼ cup raisins or dried sweetened cranberries (optional)
    ½ teaspoon vanilla

*Look for rice that cooks in 20 to 25 minutes. For rice with a longer cooking time, increase the cooking time in step 1.

1. Bring 1½ cups soymilk to a simmer in medium saucepan. Stir in rice, brown sugar, cinnamon and salt. Reduce heat to low; cover and simmer 10 minutes.

2. Stir in remaining ½ cup soymilk and raisins, if desired. Cover and simmer 10 minutes. Remove from heat; stir in vanilla.

Note: Rice thickens as it cools. For a thinner consistency, stir in additional soymilk.

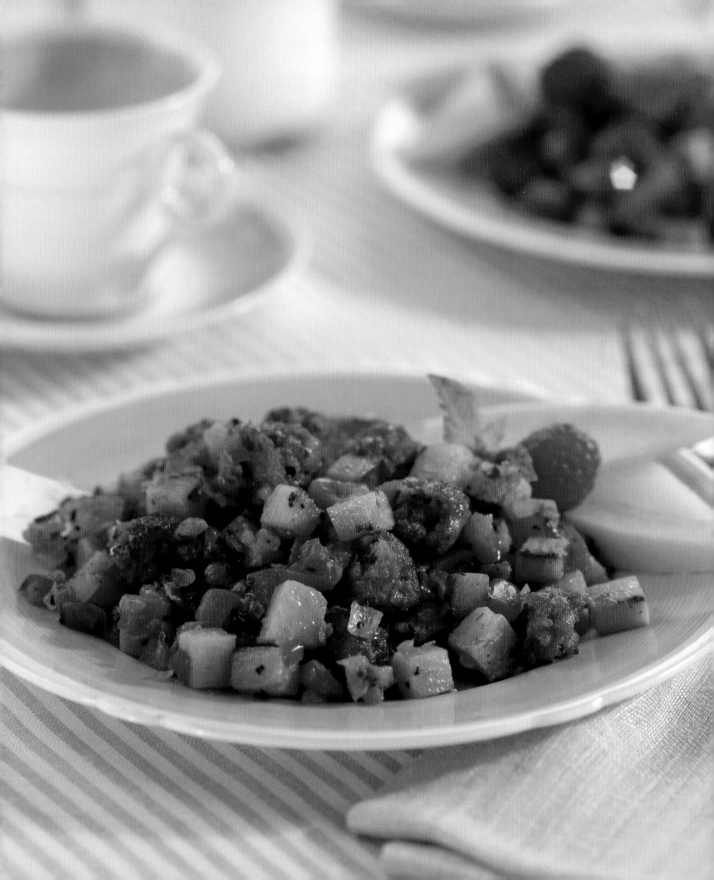

BANANA CHOCOLATE CHIP BUTTERMILK PANCAKES

Makes 24 pancakes (about 8 servings)

2½ cups Gluten-Free All-Purpose Flour Blend (page 19)*
⅓ cup sugar
1½ teaspoons baking powder
1 teaspoon baking soda
½ teaspoon ground cinnamon
1½ cups low-fat buttermilk
3 eggs
1 teaspoon vanilla
1½ cups mashed bananas (about 3 medium)
   Vegetable oil
¾ cup milk chocolate chips, plus additional for garnish
   Butter and/or maple syrup

Or use any all-purpose gluten-free flour blend that does not contain xanthan gum.

1. Combine flour blend, sugar, baking powder, baking soda and cinnamon in large bowl. Whisk buttermilk, eggs and vanilla in medium bowl. Gradually whisk buttermilk mixture into flour mixture until smooth. Fold in bananas.

2. Heat oil on griddle or in large nonstick skillet over medium heat. Pour ¼ cupfuls of batter 2 inches apart onto griddle. Place about 10 chocolate chips on each pancake. Cook 2 to 3 minutes or until lightly browned and edges begin to bubble. Turn over; cook 2 minutes or until lightly browned. Repeat with remaining batter and chocolate chips. Serve with butter and/or maple syrup. Top with additional chocolate chips.

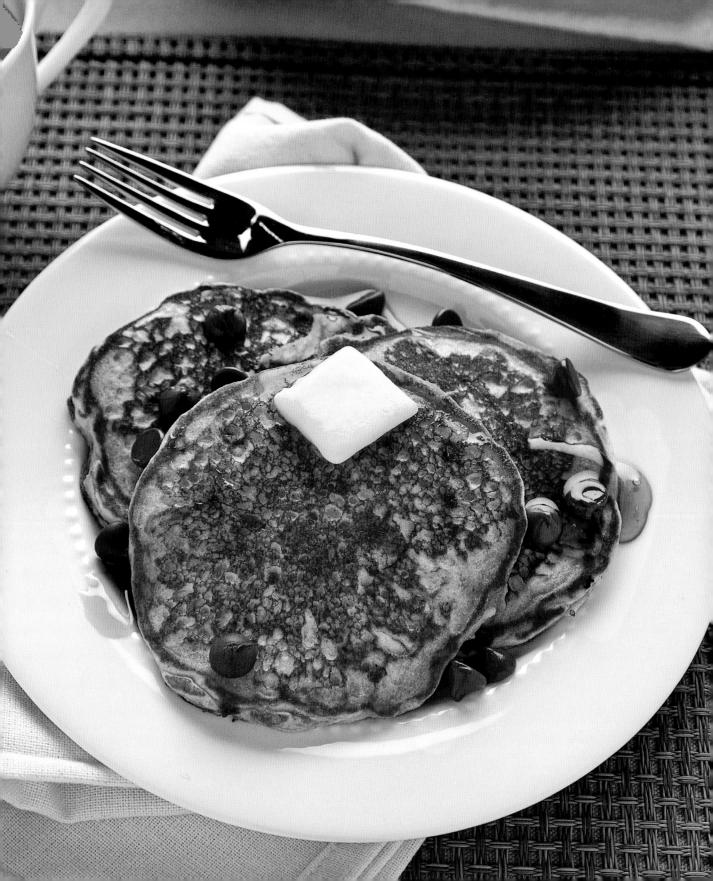

BLUEBERRY-ORANGE FRENCH TOAST CASSEROLE

Makes 6 servings

  10 slices gluten-free bread, cut into 1-inch cubes
   3 tablespoons butter, melted
1½ cups milk
   3 eggs
  ½ cup sugar
   1 tablespoon grated orange peel
  ½ teaspoon vanilla
1½ cups fresh blueberries

1. Grease 8- or 9-inch square baking dish.

2. Combine bread cubes and butter in small bowl; toss to coat.

3. Whisk milk, eggs, sugar, orange peel and vanilla in large bowl until well blended. Add bread and blueberries; toss to coat. Pour into prepared baking dish. Cover and refrigerate at least 8 hours or overnight.

4. Preheat oven to 325°F. Bake 1 hour or until bread is browned and center is almost set. Let stand 5 minutes before serving.

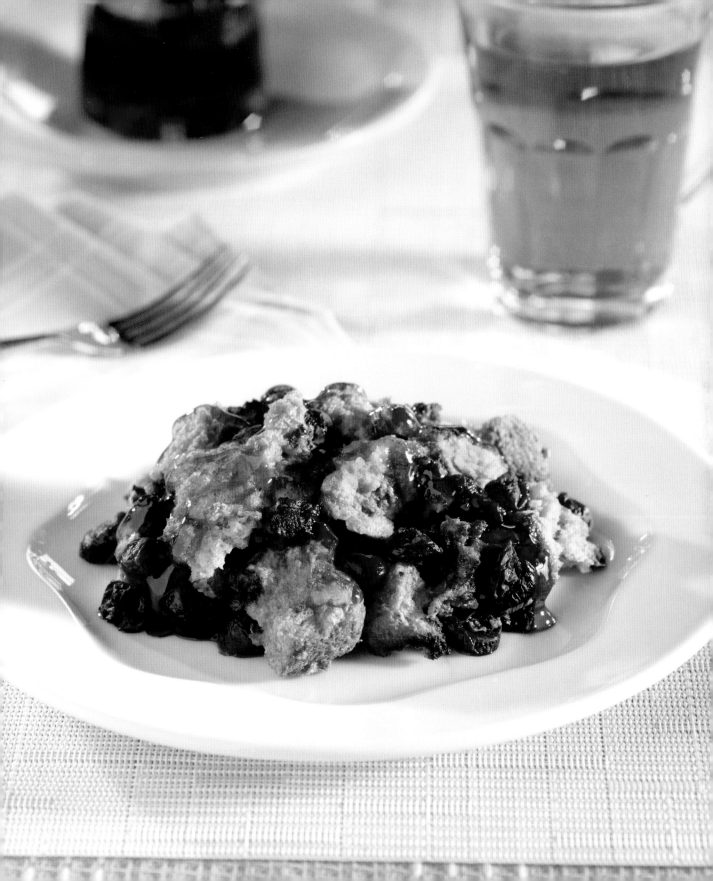

GREEN PEPPER SAUSAGE GRITS

Makes 4 servings

   2 cups water
½ cup quick-cooking grits
¼ teaspoon salt, divided
   6 ounces fully cooked turkey breakfast sausage links
   2 teaspoons extra virgin olive oil
   1 cup diced green bell pepper
   1 cup grape tomatoes, quartered
   2 cloves garlic, minced
¼ cup water
¼ cup finely chopped green onion (green and white parts)
⅛ teaspoon ground red pepper
   2 tablespoons chopped fresh parsley

1. Bring water to a boil in medium saucepan over high heat. Gradually stir in grits; reduce heat. Cover and simmer 6 minutes or until thickened, stirring occasionally. Stir in ⅛ teaspoon salt. Set aside.

2. Meanwhile, spray large skillet with nonstick cooking spray; heat over medium-high heat. Add sausage; cook until browned, stirring to break up meat. Remove to plate.

3. Heat oil in same skillet over medium-high heat. Add bell pepper; cook and stir 3 minutes. Add tomatoes and garlic; cook 3 minutes or until softened. Stir in water until well blended. Remove from heat.

4. Stir sausage and any accumulated juices, green onions, ground red pepper and remaining ⅛ teaspoon salt into skillet.

5. Divide grits among four serving plates. Top with sausage mixture and parsley.

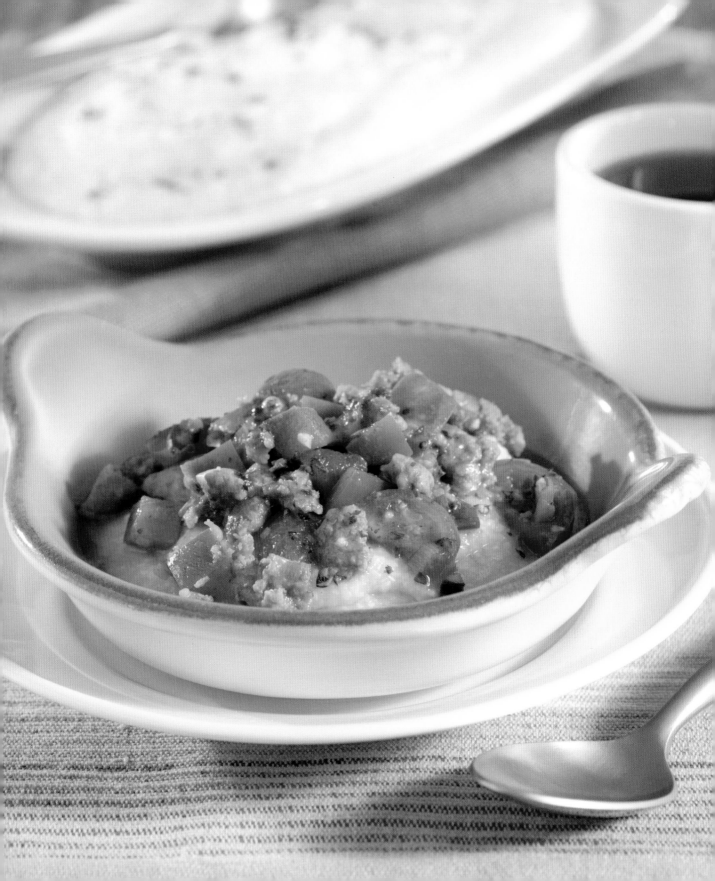

BANANA-NUT BUTTERMILK WAFFLES

Makes 4 waffles (about 4 servings)

2½ cups Gluten-Free All-Purpose Flour Blend (page 19)*
¼ cup sugar
2 teaspoons baking powder
2 teaspoons baking soda
1 teaspoon salt
2 eggs, separated
2 cups low-fat buttermilk
2 very ripe bananas, mashed (about 1 cup)
¼ cup (½ stick) butter, melted
1½ teaspoons vanilla
¾ cup chopped walnuts or pecans, toasted,** plus additional for garnish
   Maple syrup and banana slices

*Or use any all-purpose gluten-free flour blend that does not contain xanthan gum.
**To toast walnuts, spread in single layer in heavy skillet. Cook over medium heat 1 to 2 minutes or until nuts are lightly browned, stirring frequently. Remove from skillet immediately. Cool before using.

1. Spray waffle iron with nonstick cooking spray; preheat according to manufacturer's directions.

2. Combine flour blend, sugar, baking powder, baking soda and salt in large bowl; mix well. Beat egg yolks in medium bowl. Stir in buttermilk, mashed bananas, butter and vanilla until well blended. Stir buttermilk mixture into flour mixture just until moistened. Fold in ¾ cup walnuts.

3. Beat egg whites in medium bowl with electric mixer at high speed until stiff peaks form. Fold egg whites into batter.

4. Pour ¾ cup batter into waffle iron; cook about 5 minutes or until steam stops escaping from around edges and waffle is golden brown. Repeat with remaining batter. Serve with maple syrup and banana slices. Garnish with additional walnuts.

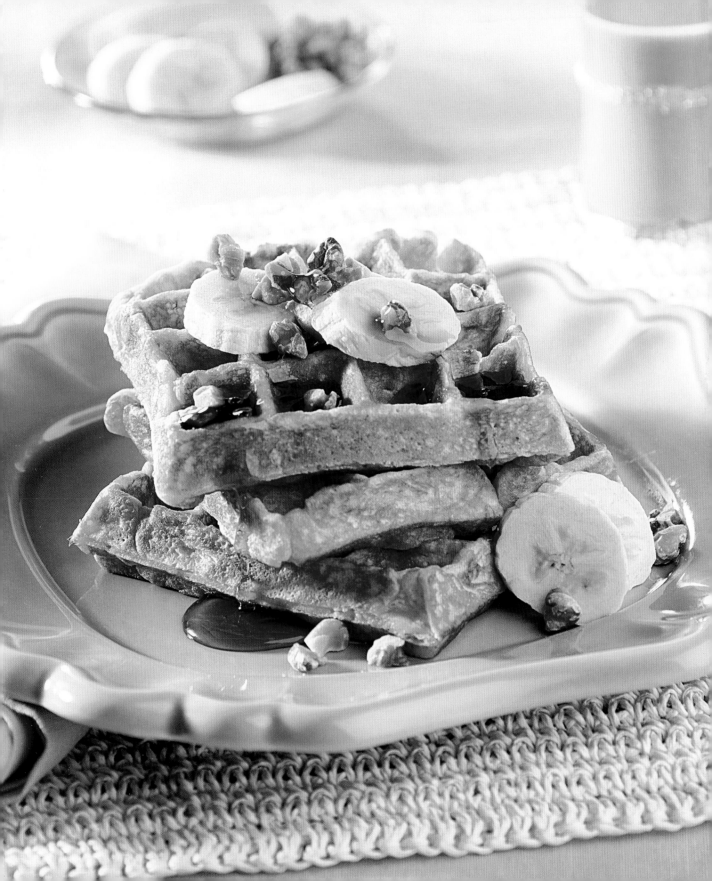

BACON & EGG BREAKFAST STRATA

Makes 8 servings

> 8 to 10 slices gluten-free white sandwich bread, cut into ½-inch cubes (about 6 cups)
> 2 cups (8 ounces) shredded sharp Cheddar cheese
> 1 package (8 ounces) bacon, crisp-cooked and crumbled
> 6 eggs
> 2 cups reduced-fat (2%) milk
> ½ teaspoon salt
> ½ teaspoon black pepper

1. Preheat oven to 350°F. Spray 13×9-inch baking dish with nonstick cooking spray.

2. Arrange bread cubes in prepared baking dish. Top evenly with cheese and bacon.

3. Beat eggs in large bowl; gradually whisk in milk, salt and pepper. Pour evenly over bread cubes, pressing down lightly until evenly coated.

4. Bake 35 to 40 minutes or until golden brown and knife inserted into center comes out clean.

BREAKFAST QUINOA

Makes 6 servings

> 1½ cups uncooked quinoa
> 3 cups water
> 3 tablespoons packed brown sugar
> 2 tablespoons maple syrup
> 1½ teaspoons ground cinnamon
> ¾ cup raisins (optional)

Slow Cooker Directions

1. Place quinoa in fine-mesh strainer; rinse well under cold running water. Transfer to slow cooker.

2. Stir water, brown sugar, maple syrup and cinnamon into slow cooker. Cover; cook on LOW 5 hours or on HIGH 2½ hours or until quinoa is tender and water is absorbed.

3. Add raisins, if desired, during last 10 to 15 minutes of cooking.

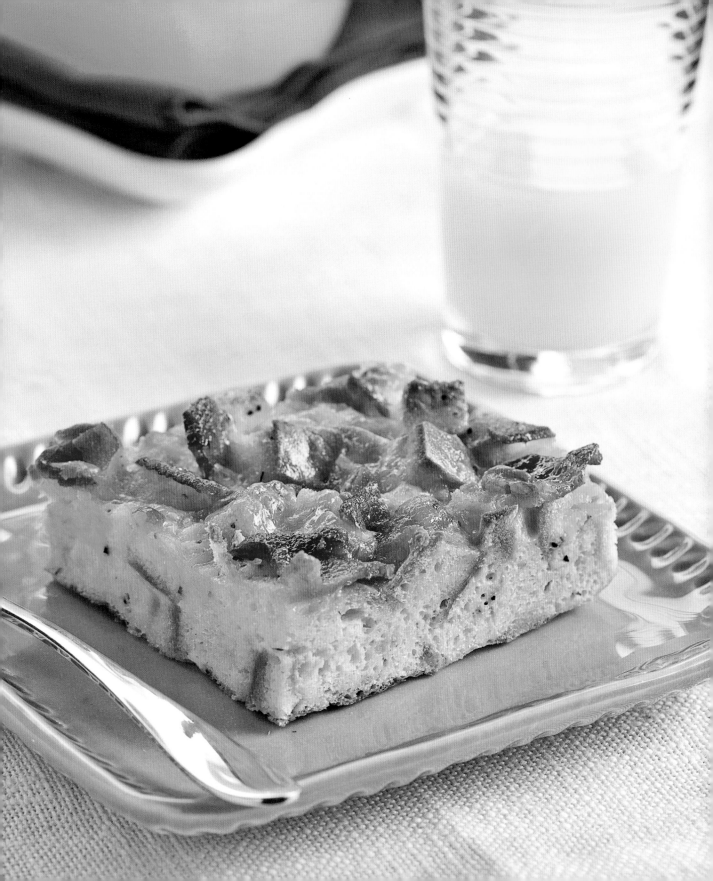

CHEESY QUICHETTES

Makes 12 quichettes

　　12 slices bacon, crisp-cooked and chopped
　　6 eggs, beaten
　　¼ cup whole milk
　　1½ cups thawed frozen shredded hash brown potatoes, squeezed dry
　　¼ cup chopped fresh parsley
　　½ teaspoon salt
　　1½ cups (6 ounces) shredded Mexican cheese blend

1. Preheat oven to 400°F. Lightly spray 12 standard (2½-inch) muffin cups with nonstick cooking spray.

2. Divide bacon evenly among prepared muffin cups. Beat eggs and milk in medium bowl. Add potatoes, parsley and salt; mix well. Spoon mixture evenly into muffin cups.

3. Bake 15 minutes or until knife inserted into centers comes out almost clean. Sprinkle evenly with cheese; let stand 3 minutes or until cheese is melted. (Egg mixture will continue to cook while standing.*) Gently run knife around edges and lift out with fork.

*Standing also allows for easier removal of quichettes from pan.

TIP

This recipe is perfect for a brunch, party or any other special occasion.
Make as many batches as you need to serve everyone.

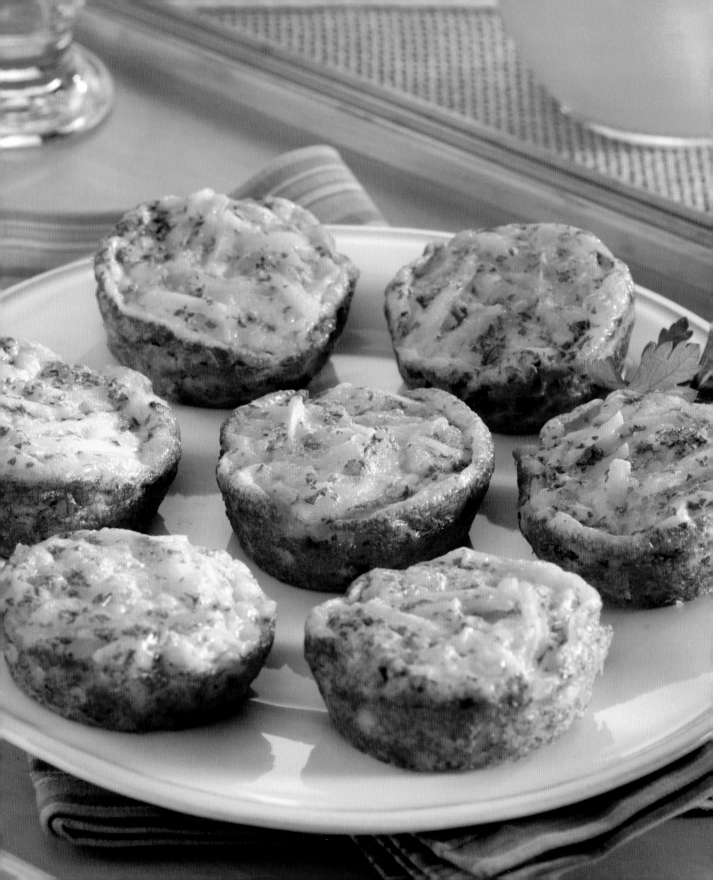

RASPBERRY & CREAM STUFFED FRENCH TOAST

Makes 4 servings

6 ounces low-fat cream cheese, softened
3 tablespoons powdered sugar, plus additional for garnish
1 teaspoon ground cinnamon
¼ teaspoon ground nutmeg
8 slices gluten-free white sandwich bread
1½ cups fresh raspberries, plus additional for garnish
⅔ cup reduced-fat (2%) milk
3 eggs, lightly beaten
2 tablespoons maple syrup
1 teaspoon vanilla
Fresh mint leaves (optional)

1. Preheat oven to 350°F.

2. Combine cream cheese, 3 tablespoons powdered sugar, cinnamon and nutmeg in small bowl; mix well. Spread evenly onto one side of bread slices. Sprinkle 1½ cups raspberries over half of bread slices; top with remaining bread slices, pressing down gently to flatten.

3. Whisk milk, eggs, maple syrup and vanilla in shallow dish. Dip sandwiches into egg mixture one at a time; let stand 5 minutes or until fully soaked. Shake off excess. Repeat with remaining sandwiches.

4. Spray large skillet with nonstick cooking spray; heat over medium heat. Add sandwiches in batches; cook 3 to 4 minutes per side or until golden brown. Place on baking sheet. Repeat with remaining sandwiches.

5. Bake 10 minutes or until bread is crisp and sandwiches are heated through. Slice sandwiches and sprinkle with additional powdered sugar, if desired. Garnish with additional raspberries and mint.

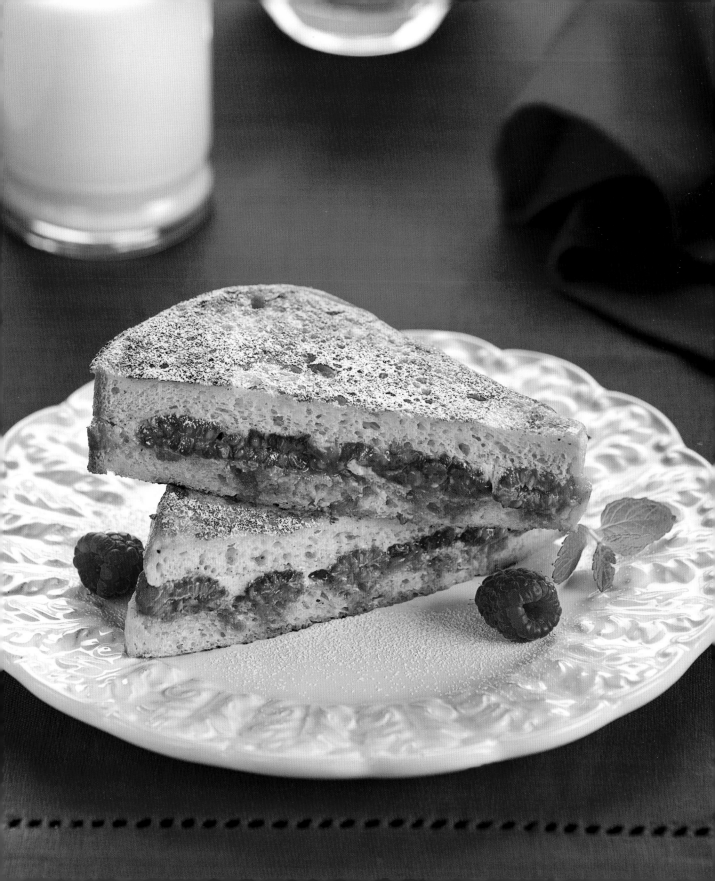

CHORIZO AND CHEDDAR BREAKFAST CASSEROLE

Makes 6 to 8 servings

    8 ounces chorizo sausage, casings removed or sliced smoked turkey sausage
    1 cup diced onion
    1 medium green bell pepper, chopped
    1 jalapeño pepper,* chopped
    6 eggs, lightly beaten
    1 cup gluten-free biscuit baking mix
    ¾ cup low-fat buttermilk
    ½ teaspoon salt
    ½ teaspoon black pepper
    1 cup (4 ounces) shredded Cheddar cheese
    ¼ cup chopped fresh cilantro
    ½ cup sour cream (optional)
    Chopped tomato (optional)

Jalapeño peppers can sting and irritate the skin, so wear rubber gloves when handling peppers and do not touch your eyes.

1. Preheat oven to 350°F. Spray 8- or 9-inch square baking dish with nonstick cooking spray.

2. Heat large nonstick skillet over medium heat. Add chorizo; cook 4 minutes or until browned, stirring to break up meat. Drain fat.

3. Add onion, bell pepper and jalapeño to skillet; cook and stir 6 minutes or until crisp-tender. Spread mixture evenly in prepared baking dish.

4. Stir eggs, baking mix, buttermilk, salt and black pepper in medium bowl until well blended. Pour evenly over chorizo mixture.

5. Bake 45 to 50 minutes or until knife inserted into center comes out clean. Sprinkle evenly with cheese and cilantro. Let stand 10 minutes or until cheese is melted. Serve with sour cream and tomato, if desired.

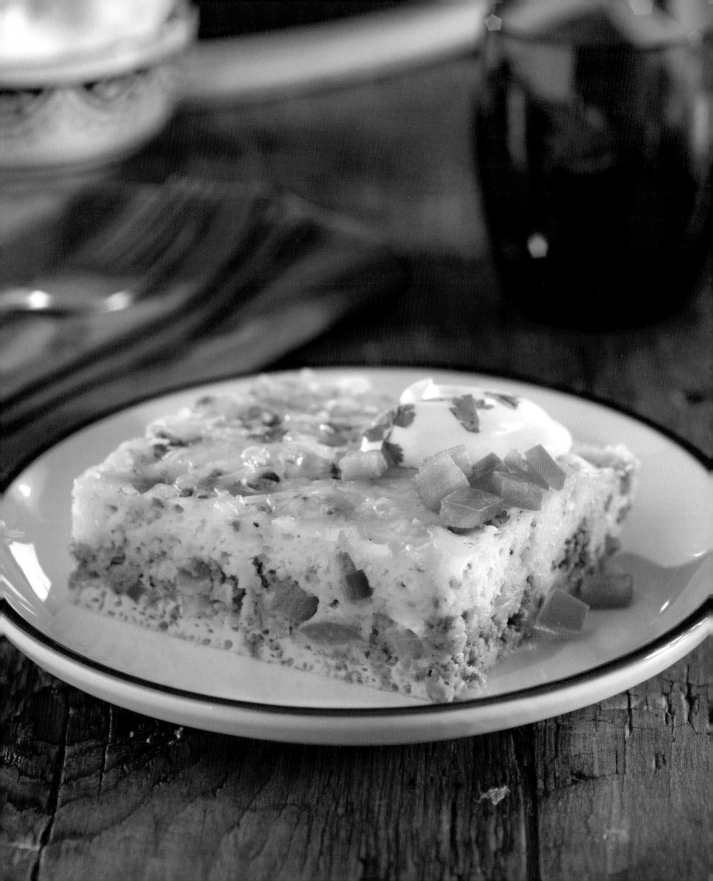

BUCKWHEAT PANCAKES

Makes 12 pancakes (about 4 servings)

> 1 cup buckwheat flour
> 2 tablespoons cornstarch
> 2 teaspoons baking powder
> ¼ teaspoon salt
> ¼ teaspoon ground cinnamon
> 1 cup whole milk
> 1 egg
> 2 tablespoons butter, melted, plus additional for cooking
> 2 tablespoons maple syrup, plus additional for serving
> ½ teaspoon vanilla

1. Whisk buckwheat flour, cornstarch, baking powder, salt and cinnamon in medium bowl. Whisk milk, egg, 2 tablespoons butter, 2 tablespoons maple syrup and vanilla in small bowl. Gradually whisk into dry ingredients just until combined. Let stand 5 minutes. (Batter will be thick and elastic.)

2. Brush additional butter on griddle or large nonstick skillet; heat over medium heat. Pour ¼ cupfuls of batter 2 inches apart onto griddle. Cook 2 minutes or until lightly browned and edges begin to bubble. Turn over; cook 2 minutes or until lightly browned. Serve with additional maple syrup.

Variation: Add ½ cup blueberries to the batter.

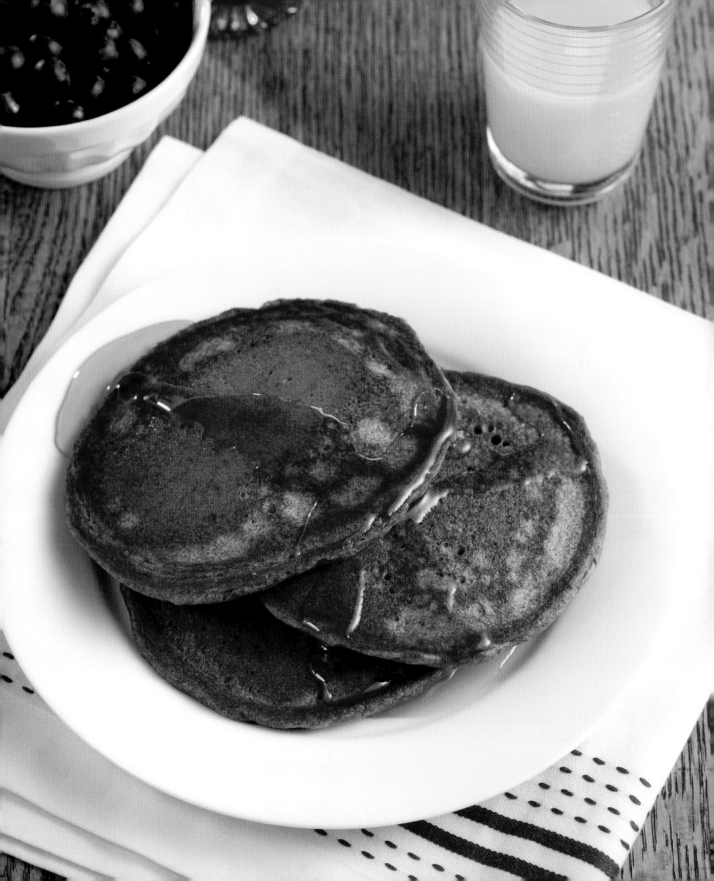

DENVER BRUNCH BAKE

Makes 4 servings

   2 tablespoons butter, divided
½ cup diced onion
½ cup diced green bell pepper
½ cup diced red bell pepper
½ cup cubed ham
  6 eggs
 1 cup whole milk
½ teaspoon salt
¼ teaspoon red pepper flakes
 4 slices gluten-free white sandwich bread, cut into ½-inch cubes
¾ cup (3 ounces) shredded Cheddar cheese, divided

1. Grease 9-inch baking dish with 1 tablespoon butter.

2. Melt remaining 1 tablespoon butter in large skillet over medium heat. Add onion and bell peppers; cook and stir 3 minutes. Add ham; cook and stir 2 minutes.

3. Beat eggs, milk, salt and red pepper flakes in large bowl. Add bread cubes, ham mixture and ½ cup cheese; mix well. Pour into prepared dish. Cover and refrigerate 8 hours or overnight.

4. Preheat oven to 350°F. Sprinkle top with remaining ¼ cup cheese.

5. Bake 45 minutes to 1 hour or until knife inserted into center comes out clean.

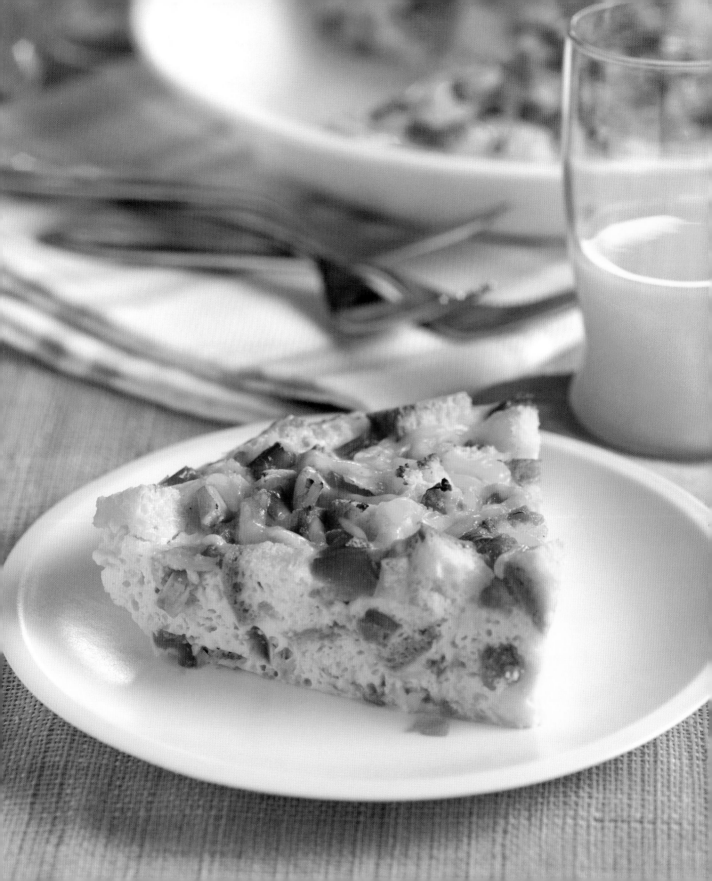

Bread Basket

YOGURT CHIVE BISCUITS

Makes 12 biscuits

 2 cups gluten-free biscuit baking mix
 1 tablespoon sugar
 ½ teaspoon salt
 ¼ teaspoon dried oregano
 ¼ cup (½ stick) cold unsalted butter, cut into pieces
 1 cup plain low-fat Greek yogurt
 ½ cup whole milk
 ½ cup finely chopped fresh chives

1. Preheat oven to 400°F. Line baking sheet with parchment paper or spray with nonstick cooking spray.

2. Combine baking mix, sugar, salt and oregano in large bowl. Cut in butter with pastry blender or two knives until coarse crumbs form. Add yogurt and milk; stir gently to form soft sticky dough. Stir in chives. Drop dough by ¼ cupfuls onto prepared baking sheet.

3. Bake 15 to 16 minutes or until light golden brown. Remove to wire rack to cool slightly. Serve warm.

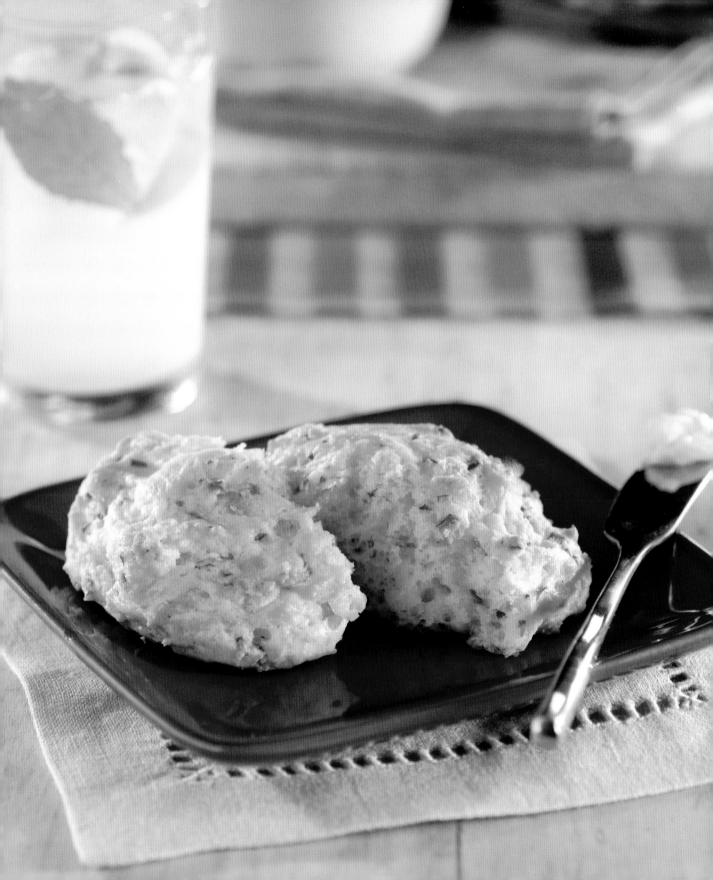

LEMON-BLUEBERRY STREUSEL COFFEE CAKE

Makes 8 servings

Streusel

    1 cup gluten-free biscuit baking mix
    1 cup packed brown sugar
 1½ teaspoons ground cinnamon
  ½ teaspoon ground nutmeg
  ½ cup (1 stick) cold unsalted butter, cubed
    1 cup chopped pecans

Coffee Cake

    2 cups gluten-free biscuit baking mix
    3 eggs, lightly beaten
  ½ cup low-fat (1%) milk
  ¼ cup granulated sugar
    2 tablespoons fresh lemon juice
    2 tablespoons unsalted butter, melted
 1½ teaspoons finely grated lemon peel
 1¼ cups fresh blueberries

1. Preheat oven to 350°F. Spray 8- to 9-inch square baking pan with nonstick cooking spray.

2. Combine 1 cup baking mix, brown sugar, cinnamon and nutmeg in medium bowl. Cut in ½ cup butter with pastry blender or two knives until coarse crumbs form. Stir in pecans. Sprinkle half of mixture evenly over bottom of prepared pan. Set remaining half aside.

3. Combine 2 cups baking mix, eggs, milk, granulated sugar, lemon juice, 2 tablespoons melted butter and lemon peel; mix well. Gently fold in blueberries. Pour batter evenly over streusel layer. Top evenly with remaining half of streusel.

4. Bake 30 to 35 minutes or until golden brown. Cool in pan on wire rack 20 minutes. Serve warm or cool completely.

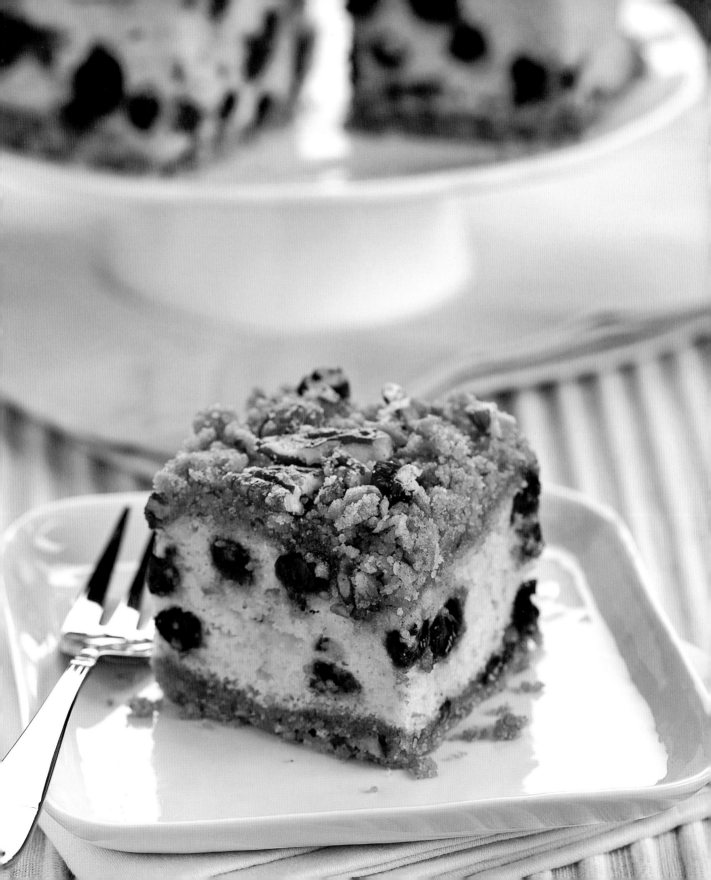

MULTIGRAIN SANDWICH BREAD

Makes 1 loaf (about 12 servings)

    1 cup brown rice flour, plus additional for pan
 1¾ cups warm water (110°F)
    2 tablespoons honey
    1 tablespoon active dry yeast (about 1½ packages)
    ¾ cup white rice flour
    ⅔ cup dry milk powder
    ½ cup gluten-free oat flour
    ⅓ cup cornstarch
    ⅓ cup potato starch
    ¼ cup teff flour
    2 teaspoons xanthan gum
    2 teaspoons egg white powder
 1½ teaspoons salt
    1 teaspoon unflavored gelatin
    2 eggs
    ¼ cup canola oil

1. Preheat oven to 350°F. Grease 10×5-inch loaf pan; dust with brown rice flour.

2. Combine water, honey and yeast in medium bowl. Cover with plastic wrap; let stand 10 minutes or until foamy.

3. Combine 1 cup brown rice flour, white rice flour, milk powder, oat flour, cornstarch, potato starch, teff flour, xanthan gum, egg white powder, salt and gelatin in large bowl. Stir until well blended.

4. Whisk eggs and oil in small bowl. Gradually beat yeast mixture and egg mixture into flour mixture with electric mixer at low speed until combined. Beat at high speed 5 minutes or until smooth. Pour into prepared pan.

5. Bake 1 hour or until internal temperature reaches 200°F. Remove to wire rack; cool completely.

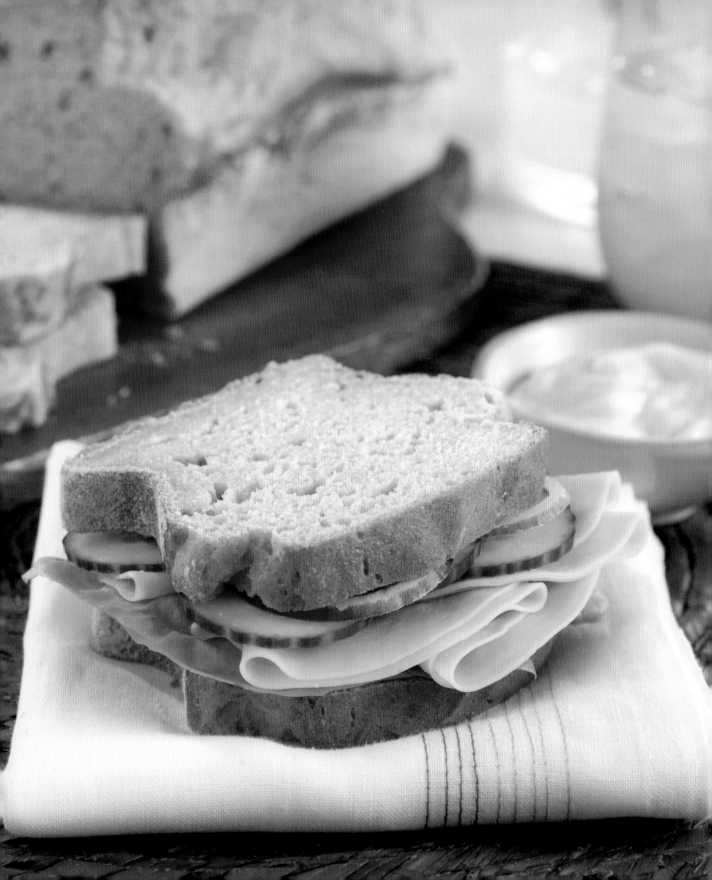

CHOCOLATE CHERRY BREAD

Makes 1 loaf (about 12 servings)

 ⅔ cup plus ¼ cup warm water (110°F), divided
 3 tablespoons sugar, divided
 1 package (¼ ounce) active dry yeast
 2 cups Gluten-Free All-Purpose Flour Blend (page 19)*
 1½ teaspoons xanthan gum
 ½ teaspoon salt
 5 tablespoons butter, melted and cooled
 3 eggs, at room temperature
 ¾ cup dried sour cherries**
 4 ounces bittersweet chocolate, chopped

Or use any all-purpose gluten-free flour blend that does not contain xanthan gum.
**If dried sour cherries aren't available, substitute other dried cherries or dried cranberries.*

1. Spray 9×5-inch loaf pan with nonstick cooking spray. Combine ¼ cup warm water, 1 tablespoon sugar and yeast in large bowl; let stand 10 minutes or until foamy.

2. Add flour blend, remaining 2 tablespoons sugar, xanthan gum and salt to yeast mixture. Whisk butter, remaining ⅔ cup warm water and eggs in small bowl. Gradually beat into flour mixture with electric mixer at low speed until well blended. Scrape side of bowl; beat at medium-high speed 3 minutes or until well blended. Add cherries and chocolate; beat at low speed just until combined.

3. Pour batter into prepared pan. Cover and let rise in warm place about 1 hour or until batter almost reaches top of pan.

4. Preheat oven to 350°F.

5. Bake 35 to 40 minutes or until toothpick inserted into center comes out clean. Cool in pan on wire rack 10 minutes. Remove to wire rack; cool completely.

Note: This bread may fall slightly after coming out of the oven.

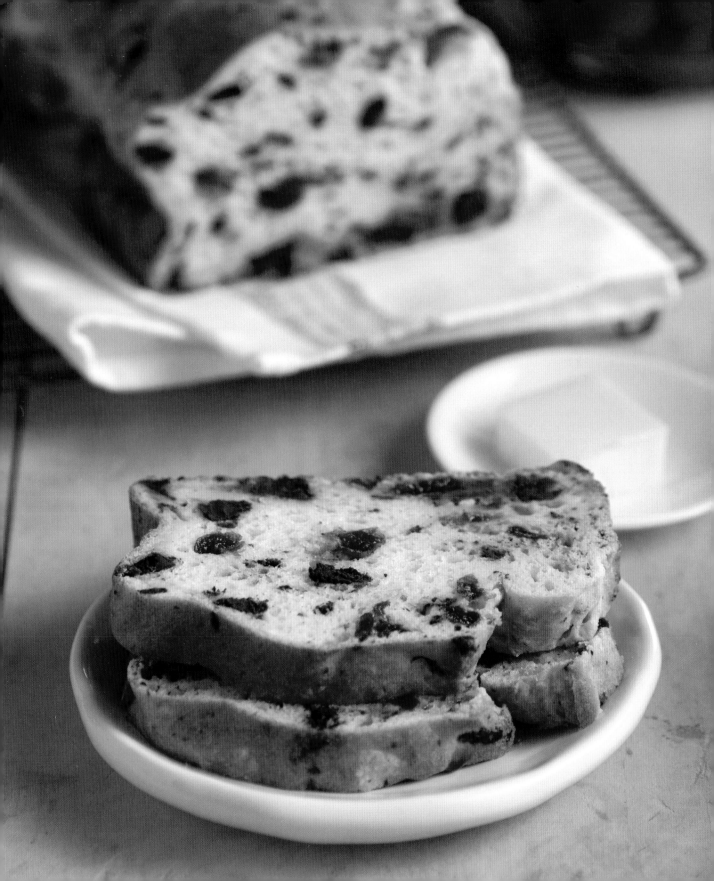

LEMON POPPY SEED MUFFINS

Makes 18 muffins

        2 cups Gluten-Free All-Purpose Flour Blend (page 19)*
  1¼ cups granulated sugar
    ¼ cup poppy seeds
    2 tablespoons plus 2 teaspoons grated lemon peel, divided
    1 tablespoon baking powder
  ¾ teaspoon xanthan gum
  ½ teaspoon baking soda
  ½ teaspoon ground cardamom
    ¼ teaspoon salt
    2 eggs
  ½ cup (1 stick) butter, melted
  ½ cup milk
    ½ cup plus 2 tablespoons lemon juice, divided
    1 cup powdered sugar
        Additional grated lemon peel (optional)

*Or use any all-purpose gluten-free flour blend that does not contain xanthan gum.

1. Preheat oven to 400°F. Grease 18 standard (2½-inch) muffin cups or line with paper baking cups.

2. Combine flour blend, granulated sugar, poppy seeds, 2 tablespoons lemon peel, baking powder, xanthan gum, baking soda, cardamom and salt in large bowl. Beat eggs in medium bowl. Add butter, milk and ½ cup lemon juice; mix well. Stir into flour mixture just until blended. Spoon batter evenly into prepared muffin cups.

3. Bake 15 to 20 minutes or until toothpick inserted into centers comes out clean. Cool in pans on wire racks 10 minutes.

4. Combine powdered sugar and remaining 2 teaspoons lemon peel in small bowl; stir in 2 tablespoons or enough remaining lemon juice to make pourable glaze. Place muffins on sheet of foil or waxed paper. Spoon glaze over muffins. Garnish with lemon peel. Serve warm or at room temperature.

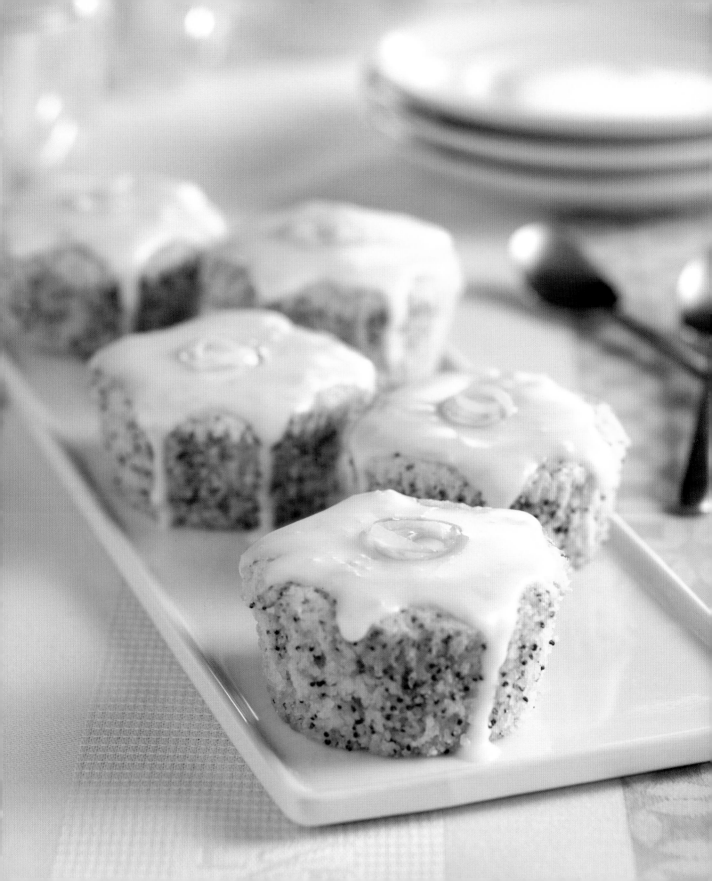

DATE & WALNUT BREAD

Makes 1 loaf (about 12 servings)

¾ cup chopped pitted dates (8 to 10 Medjool dates)
1 cup boiling water
½ cup brown rice flour
½ cup almond flour
½ cup cornstarch
¼ cup tapioca flour
¼ cup gluten-free oat flour
1 tablespoon baking powder
1 teaspoon xanthan gum
1 teaspoon baking soda
½ teaspoon salt
½ teaspoon ground cardamom
1 cup packed brown sugar
¼ cup canola oil
2 eggs
1 teaspoon vanilla
1 cup walnuts, coarsely chopped

1. Preheat oven to 350°F. Grease 9×5-inch loaf pan. Soak dates in boiling water in small bowl until dates are softened; cool slightly.

2. Combine brown rice flour, almond flour, cornstarch, tapioca flour, oat flour, baking powder, xanthan gum, baking soda, salt and cardamom in medium bowl.

3. Whisk brown sugar and oil in large bowl. Add eggs, one at a time, whisking well after each addition. Gradually stir in dates with water and vanilla. Beat into flour mixture just until combined. Fold in walnuts. Pour into prepared pan.

4. Bake 50 to 55 minutes or until toothpick inserted into center comes out clean. (Check after 35 minutes and cover with foil to prevent overbrowning, if necessary.) Cool in pan 10 minutes. Remove to wire rack; cool completely.

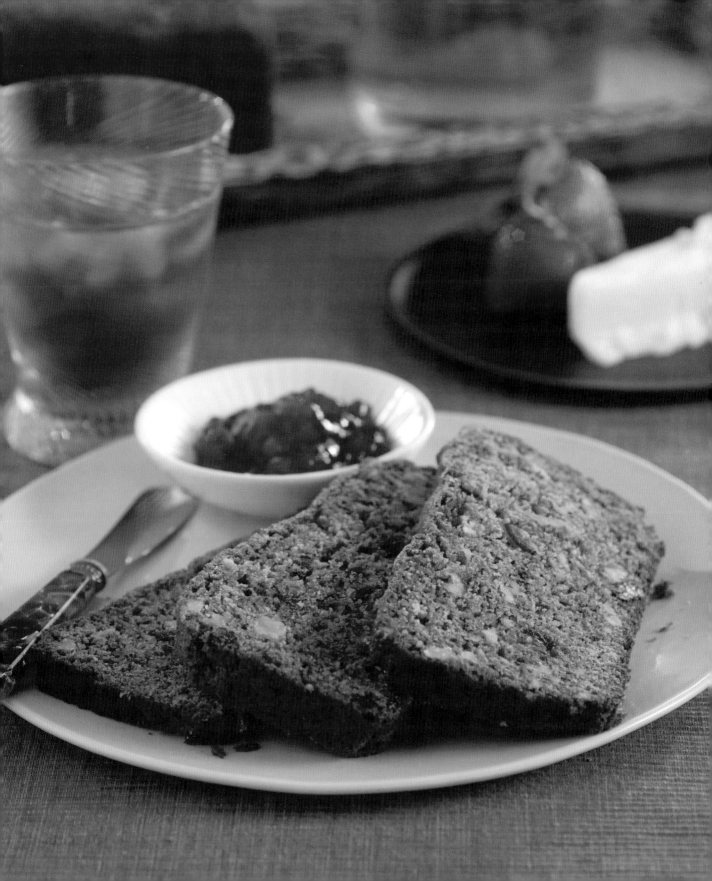

BUTTERMILK DROP BISCUITS

Makes 9 biscuits

>   2 cups Gluten-Free All-Purpose Flour Blend (page 19)*
>   2 teaspoons baking powder
> 1½ teaspoons xanthan gum
>   1 teaspoon sugar
>   ½ teaspoon salt
>   ¼ teaspoon baking soda
>   1 cup low-fat buttermilk
>   5 tablespoons unsalted butter, melted, divided

*Or use any all-purpose gluten-free flour blend that does not contain xanthan gum.

1. Preheat oven to 450°F. Spray baking sheet with nonstick cooking spray.

2. Combine flour blend, baking powder, xanthan gum, sugar, salt and baking soda in large bowl; mix well. Whisk buttermilk and 4 tablespoons butter in small bowl until well blended. Stir into flour mixture until combined.

3. Using ¼ cup measuring cup sprayed with nonstick cooking spray, drop biscuits 1½ inches apart onto prepared baking sheet.

4. Bake 12 minutes or until tops are golden brown. Brush tops with remaining 1 tablespoon butter. Cool on baking sheets 5 minutes; serve warm or cool completely.

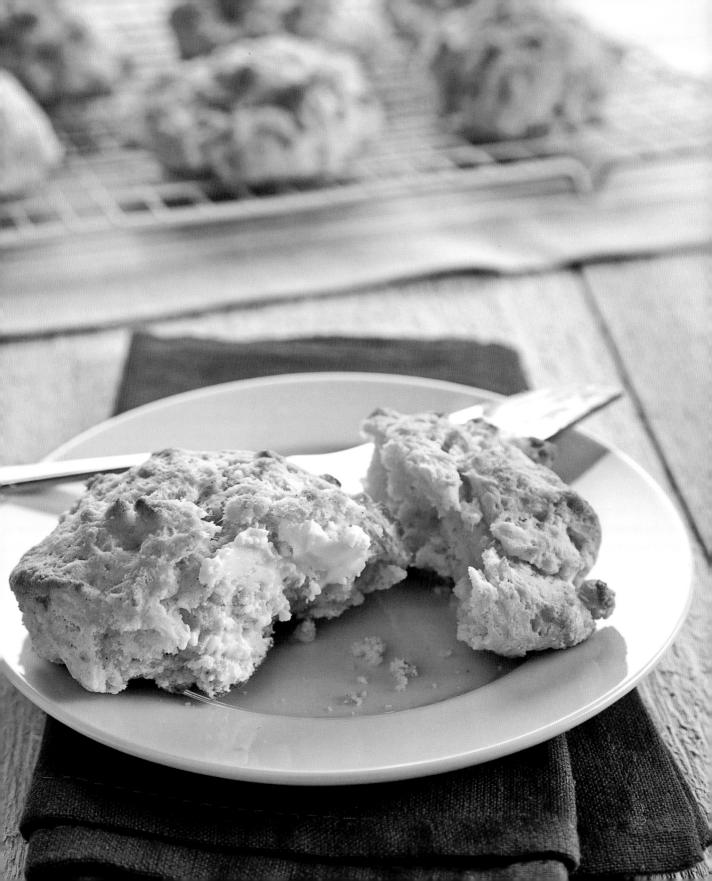

CORNMEAL PECAN MUFFINS

Makes 12 muffins

1 cup Gluten-Free All-Purpose Flour Blend (page 19)*
1 cup yellow cornmeal
1 cup sugar
1½ teaspoons baking powder
1 teaspoon baking soda
½ teaspoon salt
½ teaspoon xanthan gum
1 cup low-fat buttermilk
¼ cup (½ stick) butter, melted
2 eggs
¼ cup chopped pecans, toasted**

*Or use any all-purpose gluten-free flour blend that does not contain xanthan gum.
**To toast pecans, spread in a single layer on ungreased baking sheet. Bake in preheated 350°F oven 8 to
10 minutes or until fragrant, stirring occasionally.

1. Preheat oven to 350°F. Grease 12 standard (2½-inch) muffin cups or line with paper
baking cups.

2. Combine flour blend, cornmeal, sugar, baking powder, baking soda, salt and xanthan gum
in large bowl; mix well. Whisk buttermilk, butter and eggs in medium bowl until well blended.
Stir buttermilk mixture into cornmeal mixture just until moistened. (Batter will be thick.) Fold
in pecans. Spoon evenly into prepared muffin cups.

3. Bake 18 to 20 minutes or until lightly browned and toothpick inserted into centers comes
out clean. Cool in pan 5 minutes; remove to wire rack. Serve warm or cool completely.

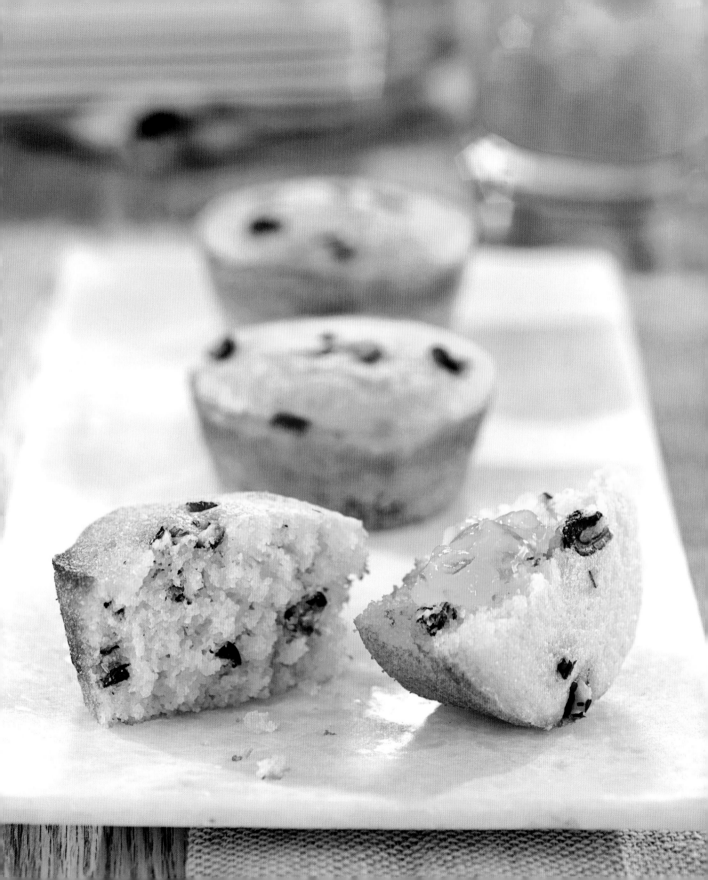

BREADSTICKS

Makes 15 to 20 breadsticks

> 3½ cups Gluten-Free Flour Blend for Breads (page 19)
> 1 package (¼ ounce) active dry yeast
> 3 teaspoons salt, divided
> 1½ teaspoons xanthan gum
> 1 teaspoon unflavored gelatin
> 1⅓ cups warm water
> 4 tablespoons olive oil, divided
> 1 tablespoon honey
> 2 to 4 cloves garlic, minced

1. Combine flour blend, yeast, 2 teaspoons salt, xanthan gum and gelatin in food processor; process until combined. With motor running, add warm water, 2 tablespoons oil and honey. Process 30 seconds or until thoroughly combined. (Dough will be sticky.) Transfer to large greased bowl.

2. Shape dough into ball with damp hands. Cover; let rise in warm place 45 minutes. Punch down dough; let rest 15 minutes

3. Preheat oven to 450°F. Line baking sheets with parchment paper.

4. Roll 1½-inch portions of dough into 8-inch-long ropes on clean work surface. Transfer to prepared baking sheets.

5. Bake 10 minutes. Meanwhile, combine remaining 2 tablespoons oil and garlic in small bowl; mix well. Remove breadsticks from oven; brush with garlic mixture. Bake 10 minutes or until browned. Remove to wire racks to cool slightly. Serve warm.

Tip: Be sure to rotate pans once during baking so that the breadsticks brown evenly.

Variation: For a sesame seed or poppy seed topping, brush breadsticks lightly with water and sprinkle evenly with seeds before baking.

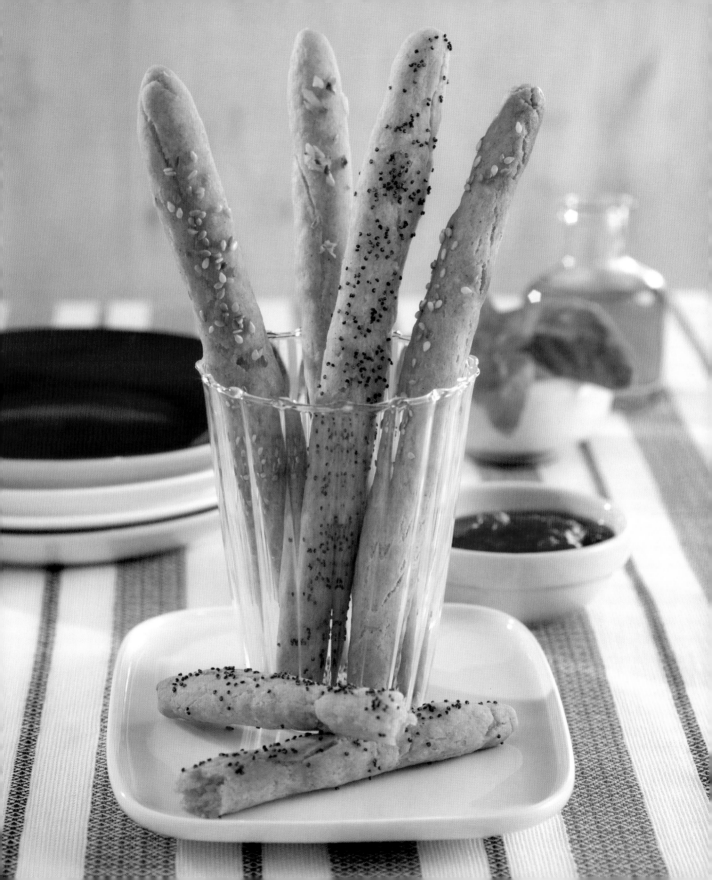

ZUCCHINI BREAD

Makes 1 loaf (about 12 servings)

2½ cups Gluten-Free All-Purpose Flour Blend (page 19)*
⅔ cup packed brown sugar
½ cup teff flour
⅓ cup granulated sugar
1 tablespoon baking powder
2 teaspoons ground cinnamon
1 teaspoon baking soda
1 teaspoon salt
¾ teaspoon xanthan gum
¼ teaspoon ground allspice
¼ teaspoon ground nutmeg
¼ teaspoon ground cardamom
1¼ cups whole milk
2 eggs
¼ cup canola oil
1 teaspoon vanilla
1½ cups grated zucchini, squeezed dry

*Or use any all-purpose gluten-free flour blend that does not contain xanthan gum.

1. Preheat oven to 350°F. Grease 9×5-inch loaf pan.

2. Combine flour blend, brown sugar, teff flour, granulated sugar, baking powder, cinnamon, baking soda, salt, xanthan gum, allspice, nutmeg and cardamom in large bowl; mix well. Whisk milk, eggs, oil and vanilla in medium bowl until well blended.

3. Make well in flour mixture; pour in milk mixture and stir just until blended. Stir in zucchini. Pour into prepared pan.

4. Bake 1 hour or until toothpick inserted into center comes out almost clean. Cool in pan on wire rack 5 minutes. Remove to wire rack; cool completely.

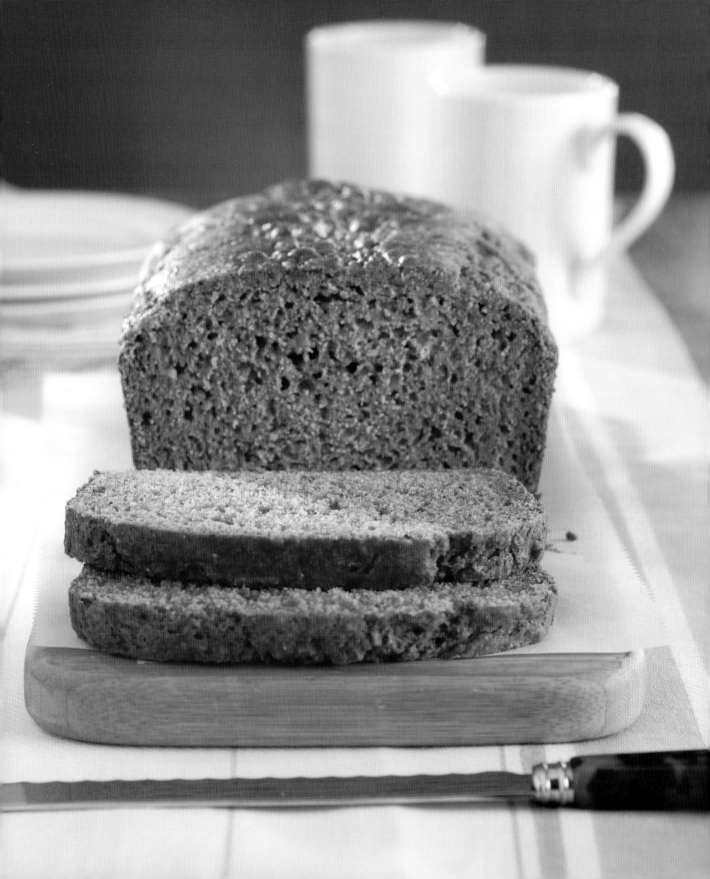

CHOCOLATE CHIP SCONES

Makes 18 scones

  2 cups Gluten-Free All-Purpose Flour Blend (page 19),* plus additional for work surface
  ¼ cup sugar
 2½ teaspoons baking powder
  ¾ teaspoon salt
  ¾ teaspoon xanthan gum
  ½ teaspoon baking soda
  1 cup semisweet chocolate chips, divided
  ½ cup (1 stick) cold butter, cut into small pieces
  ½ cup plain yogurt
  ¾ cup milk

*Or use any all-purpose gluten-free flour blend that does not contain xanthan gum.

1. Preheat oven to 425°F.

2. Combine 2 cups flour blend, sugar, baking powder, salt, xanthan gum and baking soda in large bowl; mix well. Cut butter into flour mixture with pastry blender or two knives until coarse crumbs form. Stir in ½ cup chocolate chips.

3. Place yogurt in small bowl; stir in milk until well blended. Gradually add yogurt mixture to flour mixture; stir just until dough begins to form. (You may not need all of yogurt mixture.)

4. Transfer dough to floured surface. Knead 5 or 6 times or until dough forms. Divide into three pieces. Pat each piece into circle about ½ inch thick. Using floured knife, cut each circle into six wedges Place 2 inches apart on ungreased baking sheets.

5. Bake 10 to 14 minutes or until lightly browned. Cool on wire rack.

6. Meanwhile, place remaining ½ cup chocolate chips in small resealable food storage bag; seal bag. Microwave on HIGH at 30-second intervals until chocolate is melted. Knead bag until smooth. Cut off tiny corner of bag; drizzle chocolate over scones. Let stand until set.

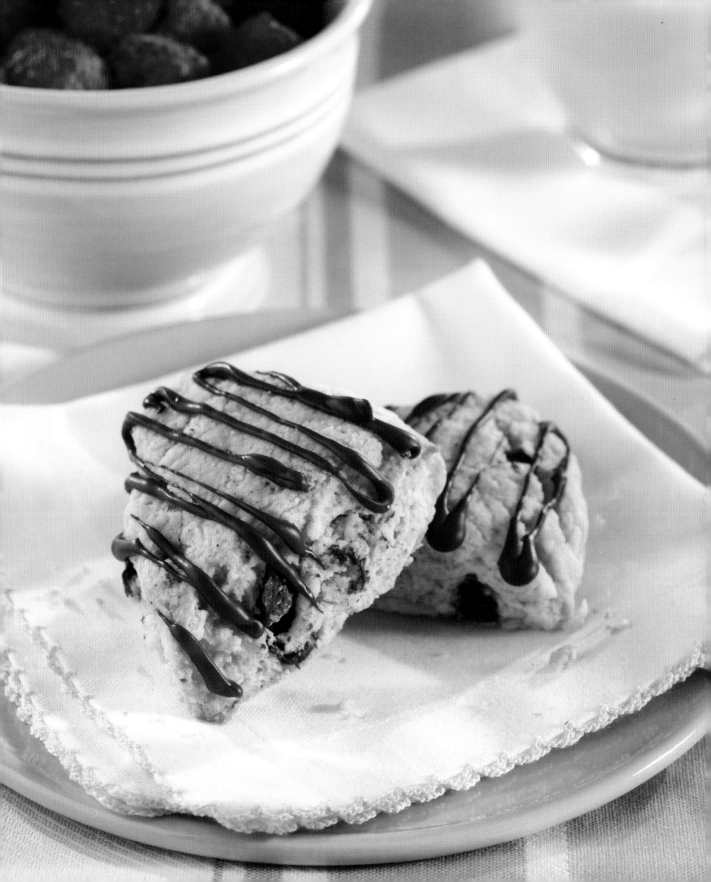

ORANGE-LEMON CITRUS BREAD

Makes 1 loaf (about 12 servings)

  1¾ cups Gluten-Free All-Purpose Flour Blend (page 19),* plus additional for pan
   ¾ cup sugar
   1 tablespoon plus ½ teaspoon grated lemon peel, divided
   2 teaspoons baking powder
   1 teaspoon xanthan gum
  ¼ teaspoon salt
   1 cup milk
  ½ cup vegetable oil
   1 egg, beaten
   1 teaspoon vanilla
  ¼ cup orange marmalade

*Or use any all-purpose gluten-free flour blend that does not contain xanthan gum.

1. Preheat oven to 350°F. Grease 9×5-inch loaf pan; dust with flour blend.

2. Combine 1¾ cups flour blend, sugar, 1 tablespoon lemon peel, baking powder, xanthan gum and salt in large bowl; mix well. Whisk milk, oil, egg and vanilla in small bowl until well blended.

3. Make well in flour mixture; pour in milk mixture and stir just until blended. (Batter will be thin.) Pour into prepared pan.

4. Bake 45 minutes or until toothpick inserted into center comes out clean. Cool in pan on wire rack 5 minutes.

5. Meanwhile, combine marmalade and remaining ½ teaspoon lemon peel in small microwavable bowl. Microwave on HIGH 15 seconds or until slightly melted.

6. Remove bread to wire rack. Spread marmalade mixture evenly over top. Cool completely before serving.

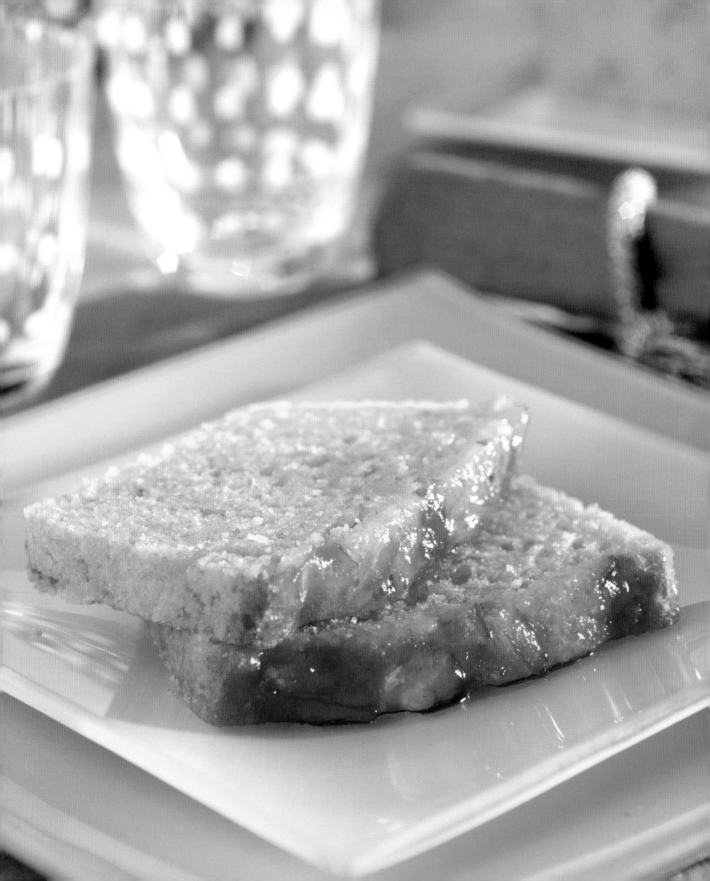

SWEET CHERRY BISCUITS

Makes 10 biscuits

   2 cups gluten-free biscuit baking mix, plus additional for work surface
   ¼ cup sugar
   2 teaspoons baking powder
   ½ teaspoon salt
   ½ teaspoon crushed dried rosemary
   ½ cup (1 stick) unsalted butter, cut into small pieces
   ¾ cup milk
   ½ cup dried sweetened cherries, chopped

1. Preheat oven to 425°F.

2. Combine 2 cups baking mix, sugar, baking powder, salt and rosemary in large bowl. Cut in butter with pastry blender or two knives until coarse crumbs form. Stir in milk to form sticky dough. Fold in cherries.

3. Pat dough to 1-inch thickness on surface lightly dusted with baking mix. Cut out circles with 3-inch biscuit cutter. Place 1 inch apart on ungreased baking sheet.

4. Bake 15 minutes or until golden brown. Cool on wire rack 5 minutes; serve warm.

TIP

Serve these sweet biscuits with jam and/or butter. They are good for breakfast, but also make a great after-school snack.

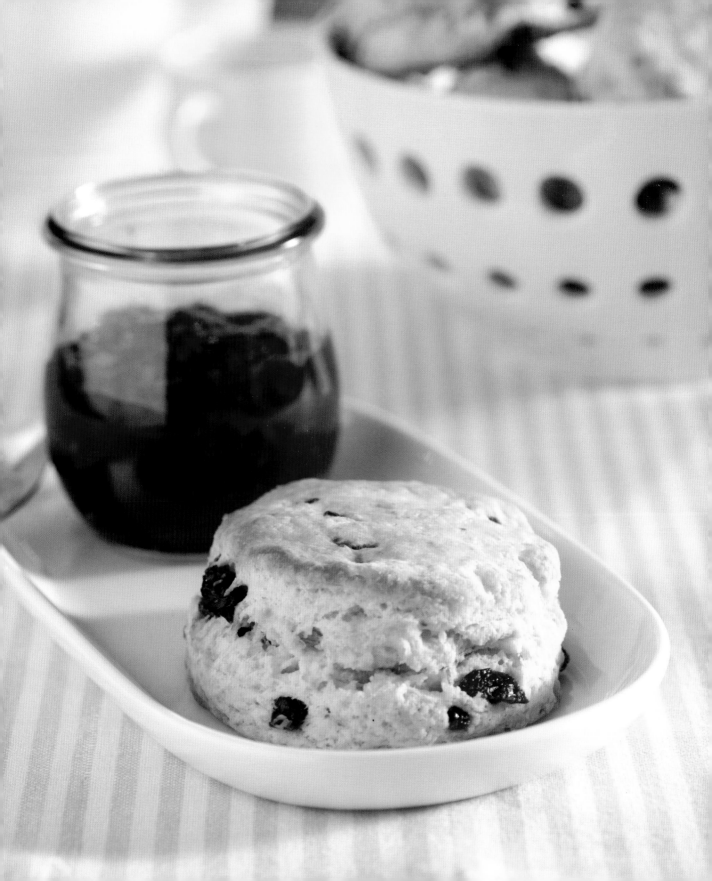

LOADED BANANA BREAD

Makes 1 loaf (about 12 servings)

  ½ cup (1 stick) butter, softened
  ½ cup granulated sugar
  ½ cup packed brown sugar
  ¼ cup sour cream
1½ teaspoons baking powder
  ½ teaspoon baking soda
1½ cups mashed bananas (about 3 ripe bananas)
  ½ teaspoon vanilla
  2 eggs
1½ cups Gluten-Free All-Purpose Flour Blend (page 19)*
  1 teaspoon xanthan gum
  ¼ teaspoon salt
  1 can (8 ounces) crushed pineapple, drained
  ⅓ cup flaked coconut
  ¼ cup mini semisweet chocolate chips

*Or use any all-purpose gluten-free flour blend that does not contain xanthan gum.

1. Preheat oven to 350°F. Spray 9×5-inch loaf pan with nonstick cooking spray.

2. Beat butter, granulated sugar and brown sugar in large bowl with electric mixer at medium speed until light and fluffy. Stir sour cream, baking powder and baking soda in small bowl until dissolved. Add sour cream mixture, bananas and vanilla to butter mixture; beat just until combined. Beat in eggs, one at a time, scraping down sides of bowl after each addition.

3. Combine flour blend, xanthan gum and salt in small bowl; mix well. Gradually add flour mixture to butter mixture, beating just until combined. Fold in pineapple, coconut and chocolate chips. Pour into prepared pan.

4. Bake 1 hour and 15 minutes or until toothpick inserted into center comes out almost clean. Cool in pan on wire rack 1 hour. Remove to wire rack; cool completely.

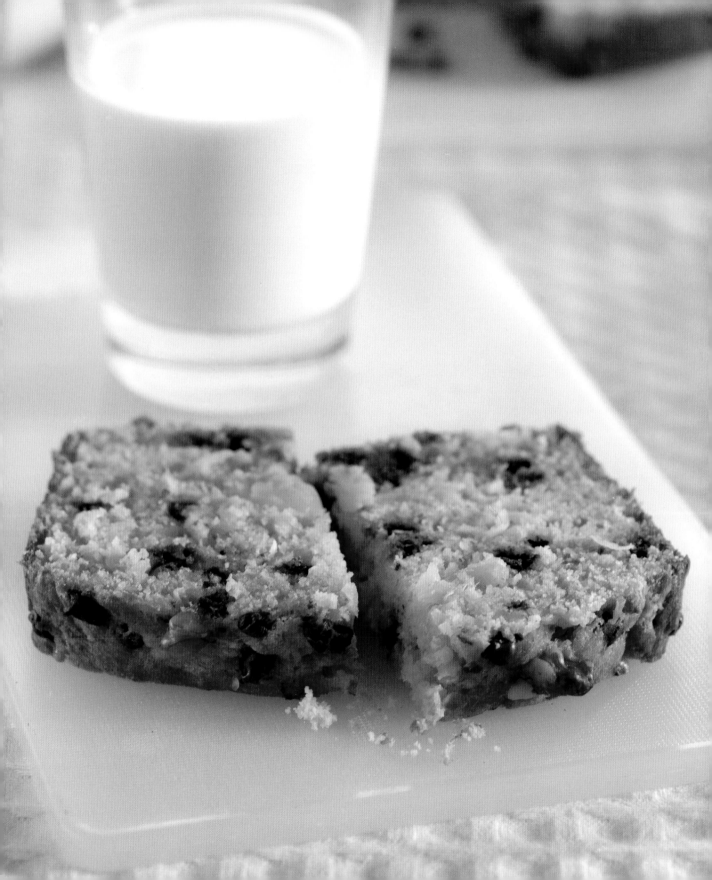

Sensational Starters

ARTICHOKES WITH LEMON-TARRAGON BUTTER

Makes 2 servings

    6 cups water
 2¼ teaspoons salt, divided
    2 whole artichokes, stems cut off and leaf tips trimmed
    ¼ cup (½ stick) unsalted butter
    2 tablespoons lemon juice
    ¼ teaspoon grated lemon peel
    ¼ teaspoon dried tarragon
    ¼ teaspoon salt

1. Bring water and 2 teaspoons salt to a boil in large saucepan over high heat. Add artichokes; return to a boil. Reduce heat to medium-low; cover and simmer 35 to 45 minutes or until leaves detach easily.

2. Turn artichokes upside down to drain well. Cut artichokes in half and remove the fuzzy choke at the bottom that covers the artichoke heart with a spoon.

3. Combine butter, lemon juice, lemon peel, tarragon and remaining ¼ teaspoon salt in small saucepan; heat over low heat until butter is melted. Serve in small bowls for dipping.

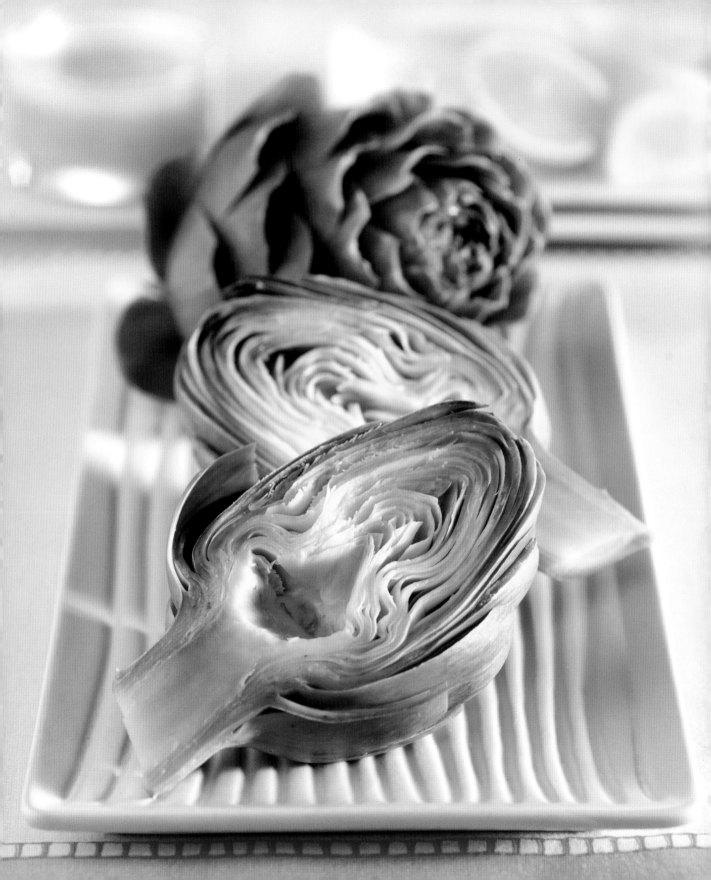

SPICY POLENTA CHEESE BITES

Makes 32 appetizers (about 16 servings)

 3 cups water
 1 cup corn grits or cornmeal
 ½ teaspoon salt
 ¼ teaspoon chili powder
 1 tablespoon butter
 ¼ cup minced onion or shallot
 1 tablespoon minced jalapeño pepper*
 ½ cup (2 ounces) shredded sharp Cheddar or fontina cheese

Jalapeño peppers can sting and irritate the skin, so wear rubber gloves when handling peppers and do not touch your eyes.

1. Grease 8-inch square baking pan. Bring water to a boil in large nonstick saucepan over high heat. Gradually add grits, stirring constantly. Reduce heat to low; cook and stir until grits are tender and water is absorbed. Stir in salt and chili powder. Remove from heat.

2. Melt butter in small saucepan over medium-high heat. Add onion and jalapeño; cook and stir 3 to 5 minutes or until tender. Stir into grits; mix well. Spread in prepared pan. Let stand 1 hour or until cool and firm.

3. Preheat broiler. Cut polenta into 16 squares. Arrange squares on nonstick baking sheet; sprinkle with cheese. Broil 4 inches from heat source 5 minutes or until cheese is melted and slightly browned. Cut squares in half. Serve warm or at room temperature.

Variation: For spicier flavor, add ⅛ teaspoon red pepper flakes to the onion mixture.

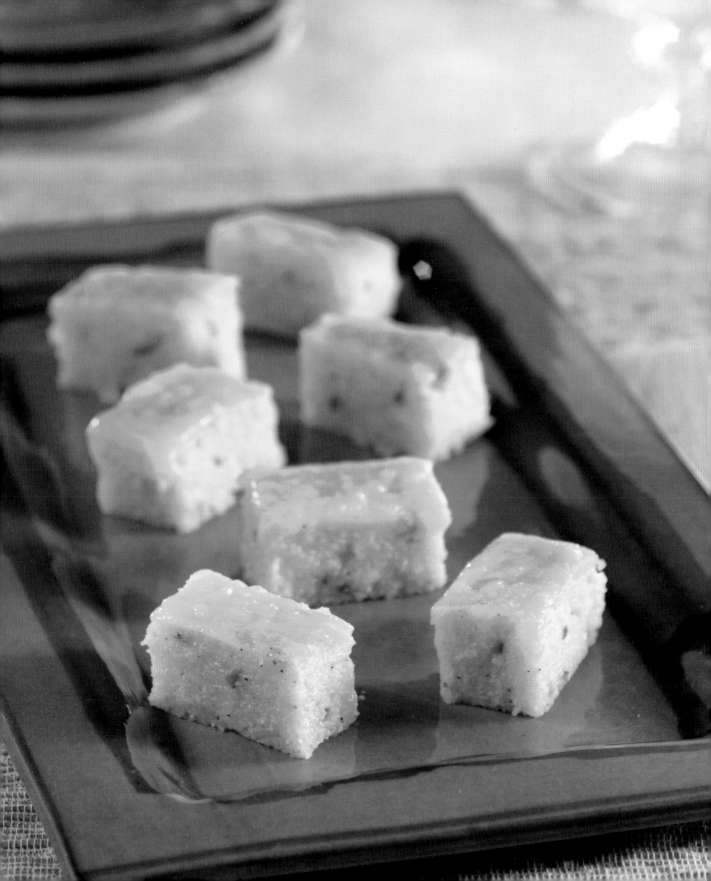

ROASTED EGGPLANT HUMMUS

Makes 2 cups (about 16 servings)

  1 large eggplant
  1 can (about 15 ounces) chickpeas, rinsed and drained
  1 clove garlic
  3 tablespoons fresh lemon juice
  2 tablespoons olive oil
  ¾ teaspoon salt
  ¼ teaspoon ground red pepper
  ¼ cup loosely packed fresh parsley, plus additional for garnish
    Assorted vegetable sticks and/or gluten-free crackers

1. Preheat oven to 400°F. Cut eggplant in half lengthwise. Place cut side down on baking sheet. Roast 35 to 40 minutes or until tender. Cool completely. Peel eggplant and remove seeds. Reserve pulp.

2. Combine chickpeas and garlic in food processor; process until finely ground. Add eggplant, lemon juice, oil, salt and ground red pepper; process until smooth. Add ¼ cup parsley; pulse until combined.

3. Serve with assorted vegetable sticks and/or gluten-free crackers. Garnish with additional parsley.

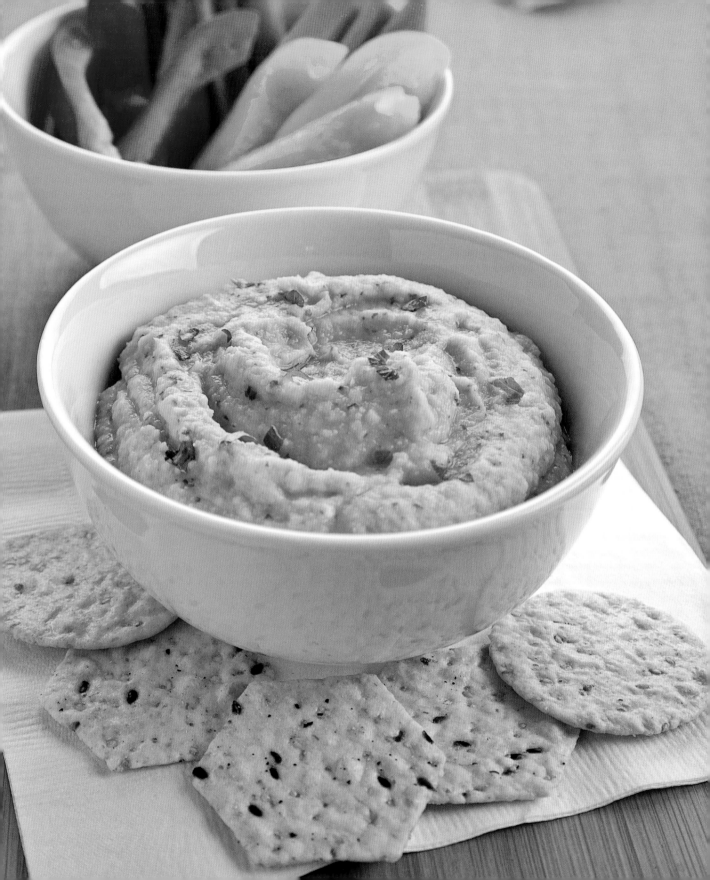

WARM GOAT CHEESE SALAD

Makes 4 servings

    1 tablespoon cornstarch
    1 egg white, lightly beaten
    ½ cup sliced almonds
    1 log (4 ounces) goat cheese, chilled
    ¼ cup sun-dried tomatoes (not packed in oil)
    ¼ cup plus 2 tablespoons olive oil, divided
    2 tablespoons balsamic vinegar
    ¼ teaspoon salt
    ¼ teaspoon black pepper
    6 cups mixed baby greens (12 ounces)
    1 cup seedless red grapes, halved

1. Place cornstarch in shallow dish. Place egg white in separate shallow dish. Place almonds in another shallow dish.

2. Cut goat cheese into 8 equal slices using thin knife dipped in hot water. Working with one slice at a time, coat goat cheese with cornstarch; shake off excess. Dip in egg, letting excess drip back into dish. Coat with almonds, pressing lightly to adhere. Place on small plate. Repeat with remaining slices. Refrigerate 15 minutes or until firm.

3. Meanwhile, combine sun-dried tomatoes, ¼ cup oil, vinegar, salt and pepper in blender or food processor; blend until smooth.

4. Heat remaining 2 tablespoons oil in medium nonstick skillet over medium heat. Add goat cheese slices; cook 2 to 3 minutes per side or until golden brown. Remove using slotted spoon to paper towel-lined plate.

5. Divide baby greens and grapes evenly among four plates. Top each serving with 2 goat cheese slices. Drizzle with dressing. Serve immediately.

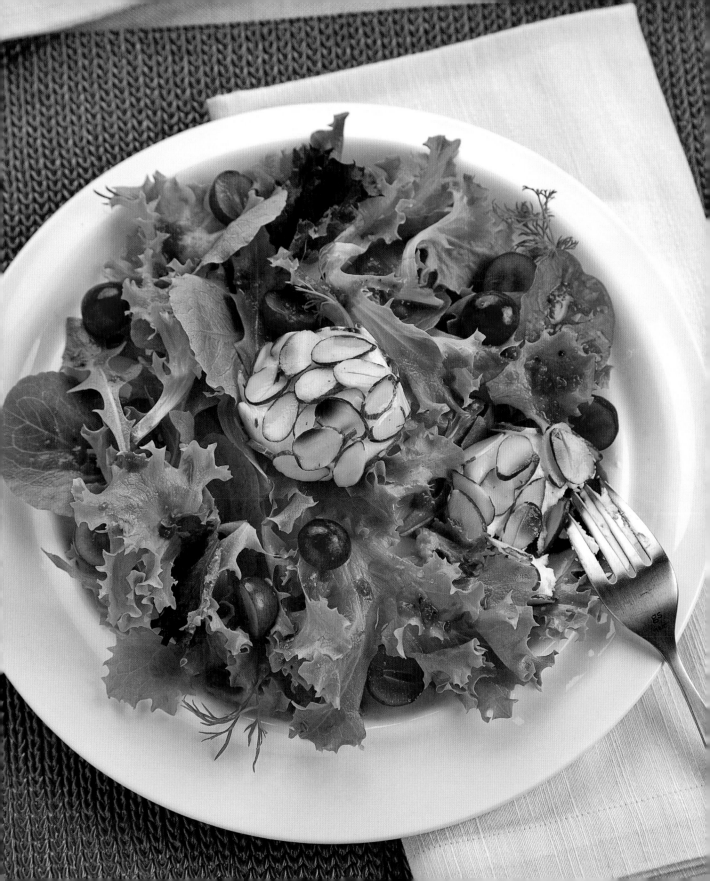

TOMATO ZUCCHINI FOCACCIA

Makes 2 focaccia breads (about 24 servings)

> **3 cups Gluten-Free Flour Blend for Breads (page 19)***
> **2 packages (¼ ounce each) active dry yeast**
> **1 tablespoon chopped fresh basil**
> **2 teaspoons xanthan gum**
> **1 teaspoon salt**
> **1 cup warm water (110°F), plus additional if necessary**
> **3 egg whites**
> **¼ cup extra virgin olive oil**
> **1 tablespoon honey**
> **1 teaspoon cider vinegar**

Toppings

> **2 plum tomatoes, thinly sliced**
> **1 zucchini, thinly sliced**
> **½ cup grated Parmesan cheese**

1. Combine flour blend, yeast, basil, xanthan gum and salt in large bowl. Whisk water, egg whites, oil, honey and vinegar in medium bowl until well blended. Gradually beat into flour mixture with electric mixer at low speed until combined. Add more water by tablespoonfuls, if necessary, until batter is smooth, shiny and thick. Beat at medium-high speed 5 minutes, scraping bowl occasionally.

2. Preheat oven to 450°F. Line baking sheet with parchment paper or foil. Transfer half of dough to prepared baking sheet. Using dampened hands or back of oiled spatula, spread into 8-inch round, about ½ inch thick. Repeat with remaining dough. Let rest 20 minutes.

3. Dimple top of dough with fingertips. Arrange tomatoes and zucchini on each focaccia, pressing lightly into dough.

4. Bake 10 minutes or until just beginning to brown. Sprinkle with cheese; bake 5 minutes or until cheese is melted.

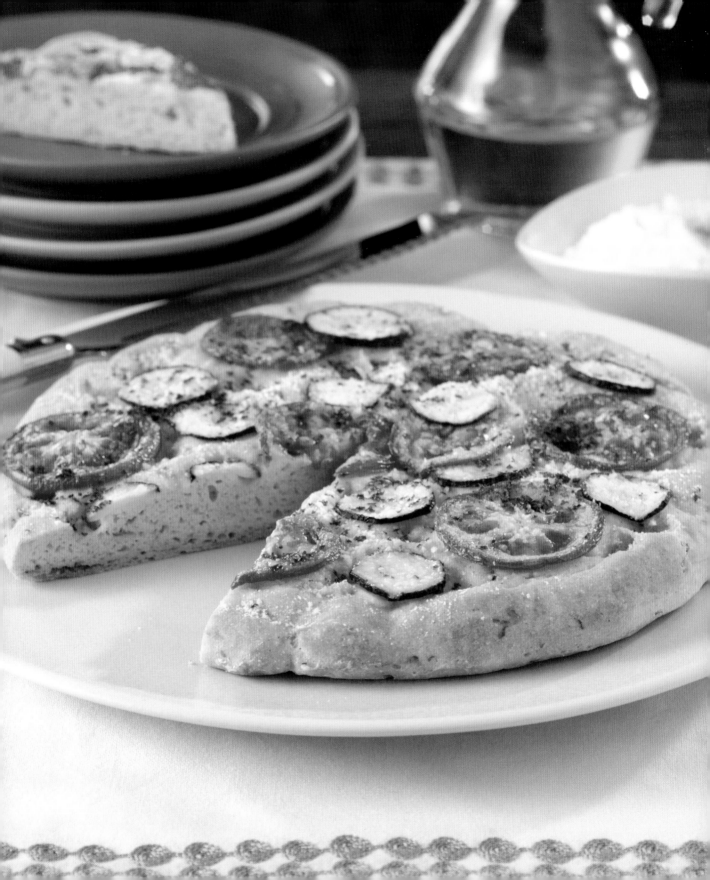

BAKED BRIE BITES

Makes 24 servings

    Gluten-Free Pie Crust (recipe follows)
  2 tablespoons walnut chips or finely chopped walnuts
  4 ounces Brie cheese
  2 tablespoons honey
  ½ cup finely chopped Granny Smith apple

1. Prepare Gluten-Free Pie Crust.

2. Preheat oven to 350°F. Spray 24 mini (1¾-inch) muffin cups with nonstick cooking spray.

3. Divide dough into 24 pieces. Roll out or pat each piece into 2-inch circle on lightly floured surface. Press dough into bottoms and up sides of prepared muffin cups. Trim edges; reroll or discard scraps.

4. Spoon ¼ teaspoon walnut chips into each crust.

5. Cut rind off Brie; discard. Cut Brie into 24 equal pieces; roll into marble-size balls. Place 1 ball in each crust over walnut chips. Drizzle each cup with ¼ teaspoon honey.

6. Bake 12 to 15 minutes or until cheese is melted and edges are lightly browned. Cool in pan on wire rack 2 minutes. Remove from pan. Top each cup with 1 teaspoon apple. Serve immediately.

GLUTEN-FREE PIE CRUST

Makes 1 (9- to 10-inch pie crust)

    1 cup Gluten-Free All-Purpose Flour Blend (page 19),* plus additional for work surface
  2 tablespoons sweet rice flour (mochiko)
1½ teaspoons sugar
  ½ teaspoon xanthan gum
  ¼ teaspoon salt
  6 tablespoons (¾ stick) cold butter, cubed
  1 egg
  2 teaspoons cider vinegar

*Or use any all-purpose gluten-free flour blend that does not contain xanthan gum.

continued on page 94

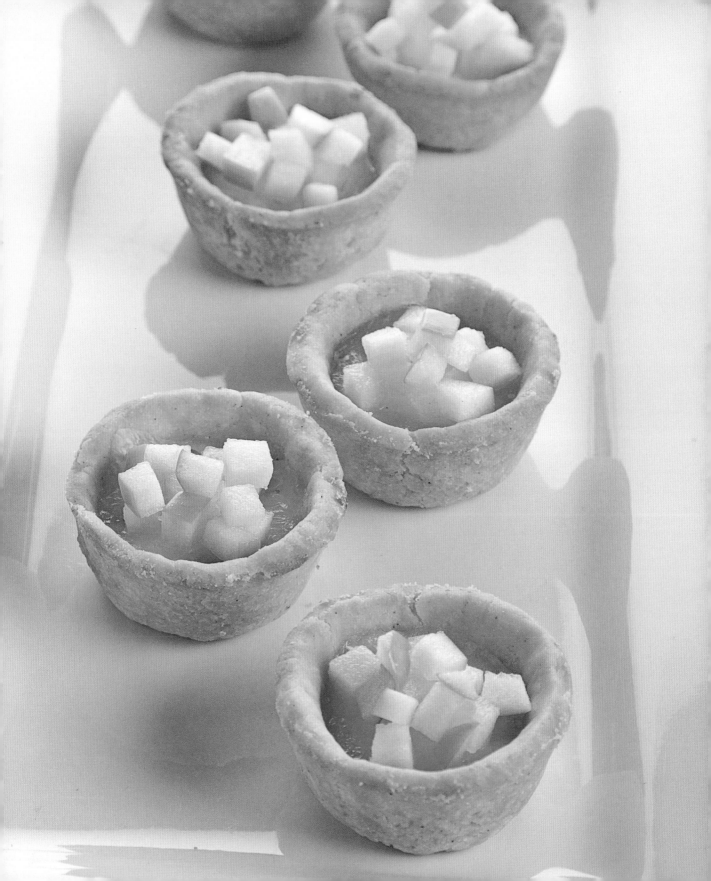

Baked Brie Bites, continued

1. Combine 1 cup flour blend, sweet rice flour, sugar, xanthan gum and salt in medium bowl; mix well. Cut in butter with pastry blender or two knives until coarse crumbs form.

2. Make well in center of mixture. Add egg and vinegar and stir just until dough forms. Shape dough into flat disc. Wrap in plastic wrap and refrigerate at least 45 minutes or until very cold.

3. Roll out dough on floured surface into rectangle. (If dough becomes sticky, return to refrigerator until cold.) Wrap in plastic wrap and refrigerate until ready to use.

QUINOA-STUFFED TOMATOES

Makes 8 servings

   ½ cup uncooked quinoa
   1 cup water
   ½ teaspoon salt, divided
   1 tablespoon olive oil
   1 red bell pepper, chopped
   ⅓ cup chopped green onions
   ⅛ teaspoon black pepper
   ⅛ teaspoon dried thyme
   1 tablespoon butter
   8 plum tomatoes,* halved lengthwise, seeded, hollowed out

Or substitute 4 medium tomatoes.

1. Preheat oven to 325°F. Place quinoa in fine-mesh strainer; rinse well under cold running water. Bring 1 cup water and ¼ teaspoon salt to a boil in small saucepan; stir in quinoa. Cover and reduce heat to low; simmer 12 to 14 minutes or until quinoa is tender and water is absorbed.

2. Heat oil in large skillet over medium-high heat. Add bell pepper; cook and stir 7 to 10 minutes or until tender. Stir in quinoa, green onions, remaining ¼ teaspoon salt, black pepper and thyme. Add butter; stir until melted. Remove from heat.

3. Arrange tomato halves in 13×9-inch baking dish. Fill with quinoa mixture.

4. Bake 15 to 20 minutes or until tomatoes are tender.

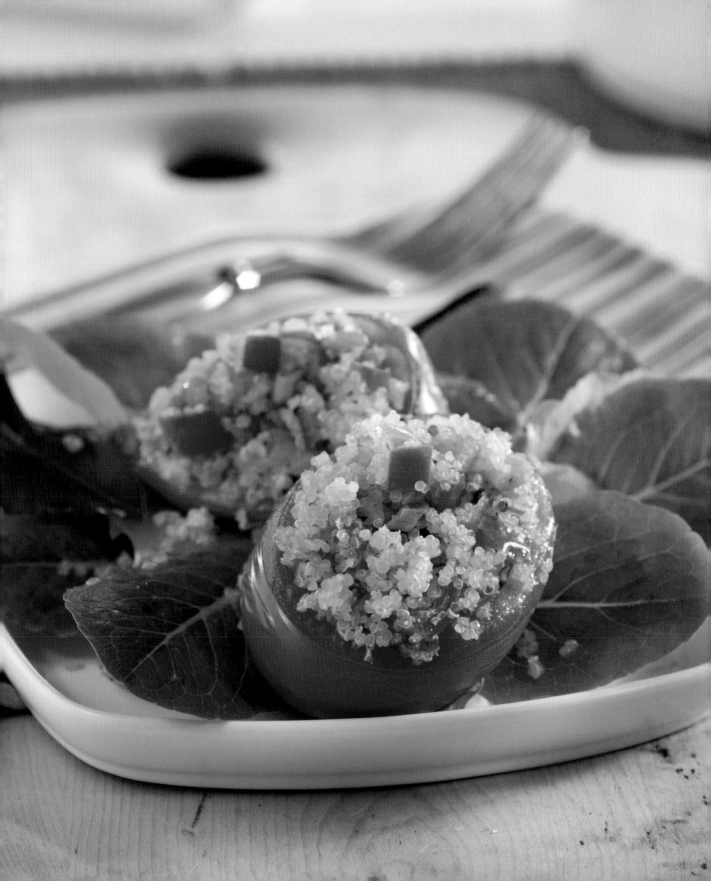

FALAFEL NUGGETS

Makes 12 servings

Sauce
   2½ cups gluten-free tomato sauce
   ⅓ cup tomato paste
   2 tablespoons lemon juice
   2 teaspoons sugar
   1 teaspoon onion powder
   ½ teaspoon salt

Falafel
   2 cans (about 15 ounces each) chickpeas, rinsed and drained
   ½ cup rice flour
   ½ cup chopped fresh parsley
   1 egg
   ¼ cup minced onion
   3 tablespoons lemon juice
   2 tablespoons minced garlic
   2 teaspoons ground cumin
   ½ teaspoon salt
   ½ teaspoon ground red pepper or red pepper flakes
   ½ cup canola oil

1. For sauce, combine tomato sauce, tomato paste, 2 tablespoons lemon juice, sugar, onion powder and ½ teaspoon salt in medium saucepan. Simmer over medium-low heat 20 minutes or until heated through. Cover and keep warm until ready to serve.

2. Preheat oven to 400°F. Spray baking sheet with nonstick cooking spray.

3. For falafel, combine chickpeas, rice flour, parsley, egg, minced onion, 3 tablespoons lemon juice, garlic, cumin, ½ teaspoon salt and ground red pepper in food processor or blender; process until well blended. Shape mixture into 1-inch balls.

4. Heat oil in large nonstick skillet over medium-high heat. Fry falafel in batches until browned. Remove from skillet using slotted spoon and place 2 inches apart on prepared baking sheet.

5. Bake 8 to 10 minutes. Serve with warm sauce for dipping.

Tip: Falafel can also be baked completely. Skip frying the falafel in oil in step 4. Instead, spray them lightly with nonstick cooking spray and bake 15 to 20 minutes, turning once.

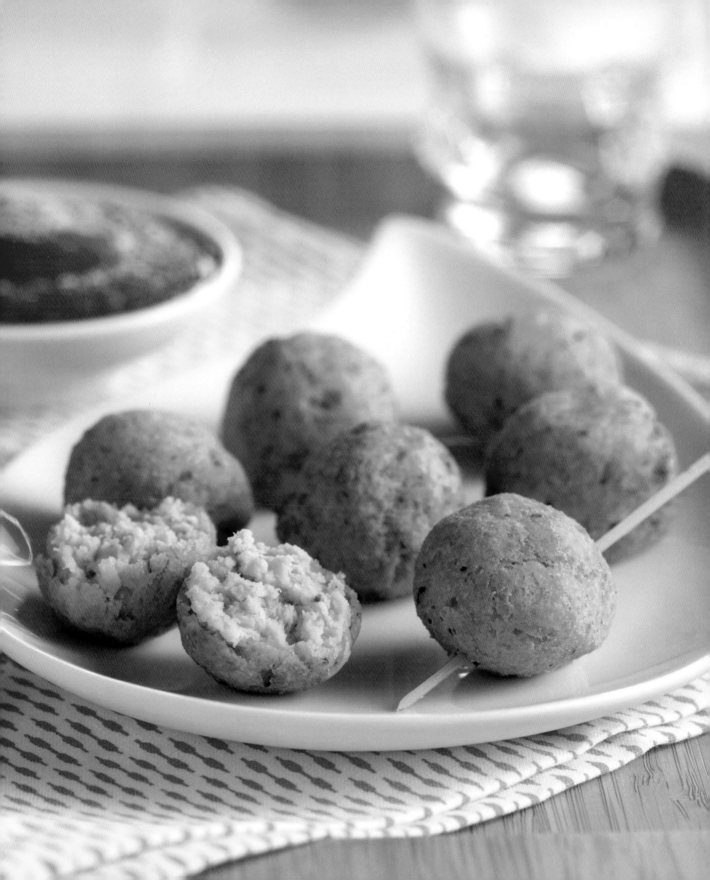

BEET AND BLUE SALAD

Makes 4 servings

    1 package (6 ounces) baby spinach
    1 cup sliced beets
    ½ cup diced red onion
    ½ cup matchstick carrots
    ¼ cup balsamic vinegar
    2 tablespoons canola oil
    2 tablespoons pure maple syrup
    ¼ teaspoon salt
    ⅛ teaspoon red pepper flakes
    ¼ cup crumbled blue cheese

1. Divide spinach equally among four salad plates. Top evenly with beets, onion and carrots.

2. Whisk vinegar, oil, maple syrup, salt and red pepper flakes in small bowl until smooth and well blended. Drizzle dressing over salad. Sprinkle evenly with cheese.

SPICY ALMOND CHICKEN WINGS

Makes about 2½ dozen wings (6 to 8 servings)

    3 pounds chicken drummettes
    3 tablespoons vegetable oil
    2 tablespoons jerk seasoning
    ½ teaspoon salt
    1 cup slivered almonds, finely chopped

1. Place drummettes in large bowl. Add oil, jerk seasoning and salt; toss to coat. Cover and refrigerate 20 to 30 minutes.

2. Preheat oven to 400°F. Line large baking sheet with foil. Spray with nonstick cooking spray.

3. Place almonds in shallow bowl. Roll drummettes in almonds until coated. Place on prepared baking sheet.

4. Bake 30 to 35 minutes or until chicken is cooked through (165°F).

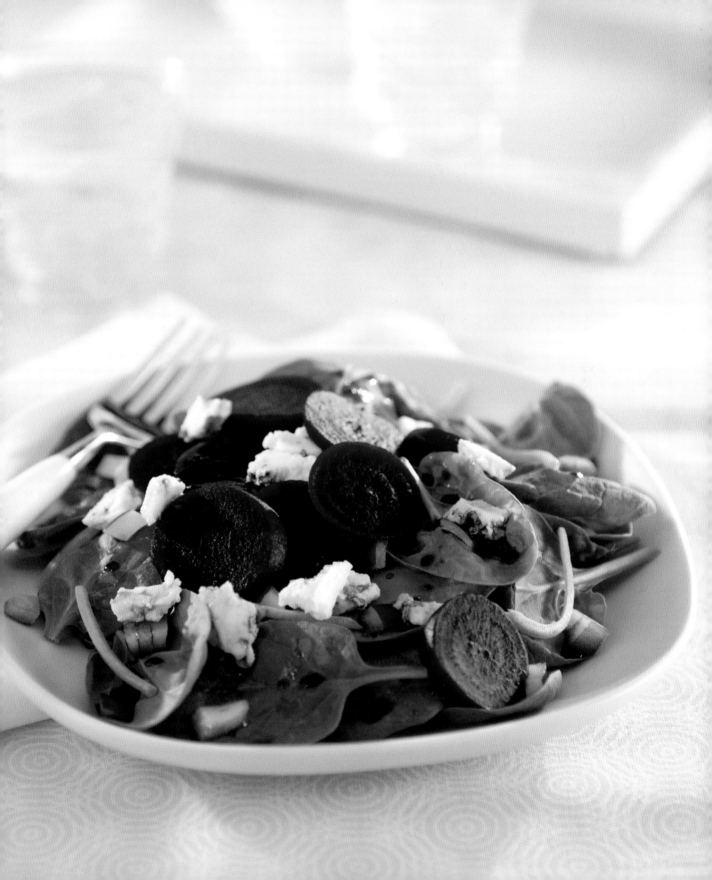

COCONUT SHRIMP WITH PEAR CHUTNEY

Makes 4 servings

>   **Pear Chutney (recipe follows)**
> ½ cup shredded unsweetened coconut
> ¾ teaspoon curry powder
> ½ teaspoon salt
> 3 tablespoons unsalted butter, melted
> 1 pound large raw shrimp, peeled and deveined

1. Prepare Pear Chutney; set aside. Preheat oven to 425°F. Spray baking sheet with nonstick cooking spray.

2. Combine coconut, curry powder and salt in shallow dish. Toss shrimp with melted butter to coat. Dip shrimp in coconut mixture, pressing lightly to adhere. Place on prepared baking sheet.

3. Bake 4 minutes. Turn over; bake 2 minutes or until shrimp are pink and opaque. Serve with Pear Chutney.

PEAR CHUTNEY

Makes 2 cups

> 1 tablespoon vegetable oil
> 1 jalapeño pepper*, seeded and minced
> 1 small shallot, minced
> 1 teaspoon grated fresh ginger
> 1 medium unpeeled ripe pear, cored and cut into ½-inch pieces
> 2 teaspoons cider vinegar
> 1 teaspoon packed brown sugar
> ⅛ teaspoon salt
> 1 tablespoon water, plus more if necessary
> 1 tablespoon chopped green onion

Jalapeño peppers can sting and irritate the skin, so wear rubber gloves when handling peppers and do not touch your eyes.

1. Heat oil in medium saucepan over low heat. Add jalapeño, shallot and ginger; cook and stir 3 minutes or until shallot is tender.

2. Add pear, vinegar, brown sugar and salt. Stir in water. Cover and cook over low heat 15 minutes or until pear is tender, adding additional 1 tablespoon water if mixture becomes dry. Stir in green onion; cook 1 minute. Cool completely.

Coconut Shrimp with Pear Chutney

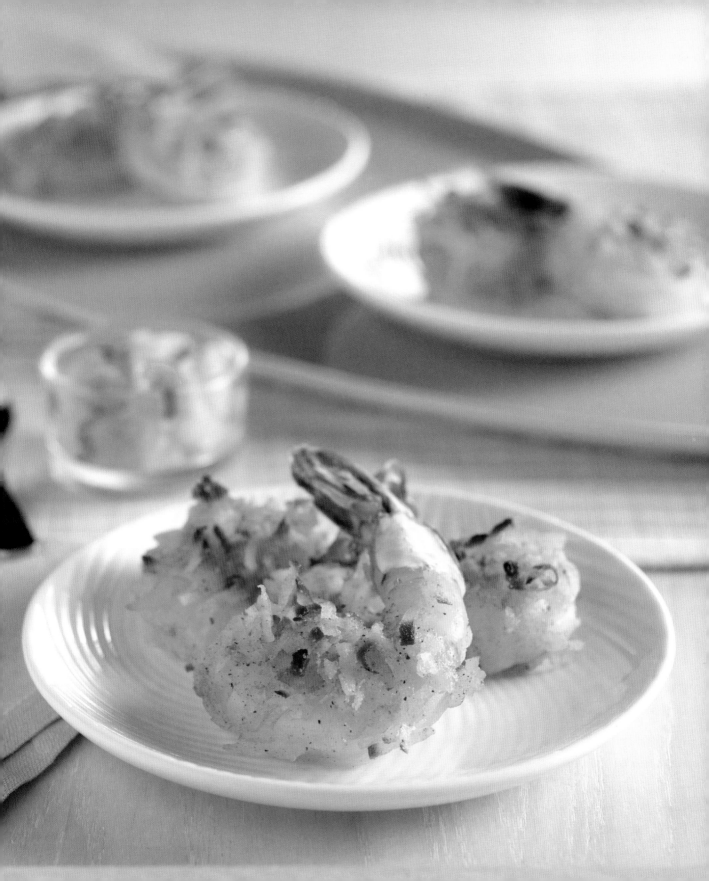

VIETNAMESE SUMMER ROLLS

Makes 12 rolls (about 6 servings)

Vietnamese Dipping Sauce (recipe follows)
3½ ounces thin rice noodles (rice vermicelli)
8 ounces medium raw shrimp, peeled and deveined
12 (6½-inch) rice paper wrappers
36 whole fresh cilantro leaves
4 ounces roast pork or beef, sliced ⅛ inch thick
1 tablespoon chopped peanuts
Grated lime peel (optional)

1. Prepare Vietnamese Dipping Sauce; set aside.

2. Place rice noodles in medium bowl. Cover with hot water; let stand 15 minutes or until tender. Drain; cut noodles into 3-inch lengths.

3. Meanwhile, bring large saucepan of water to a boil over high heat. Add shrimp; simmer 1 to 2 minutes or until shrimp are pink and opaque. Remove with slotted spoon to small bowl. When cool enough to handle, slice in half lengthwise.

4. Working with one or two at a time, soften rice paper wrappers in large bowl of warm water 30 to 40 seconds or until pliable. Drain on paper towels and transfer to clean work surface. Arrange 3 cilantro leaves in center of wrapper. Layer with 2 shrimp halves, pork and rice noodles.

5. Fold bottom of wrapper up over filling; fold in each side and roll up to enclose filling. Repeat with remaining wrappers. Sprinkle with peanuts; garnish with lime peel. Serve with Vietnamese Dipping Sauce.

VIETNAMESE DIPPING SAUCE

Makes about 1 cup

½ cup water
¼ cup gluten-free fish sauce
2 tablespoons lime juice
1 tablespoon sugar
1 clove garlic, minced
¼ teaspoon chili oil

Combine all ingredients in small bowl; mix well.

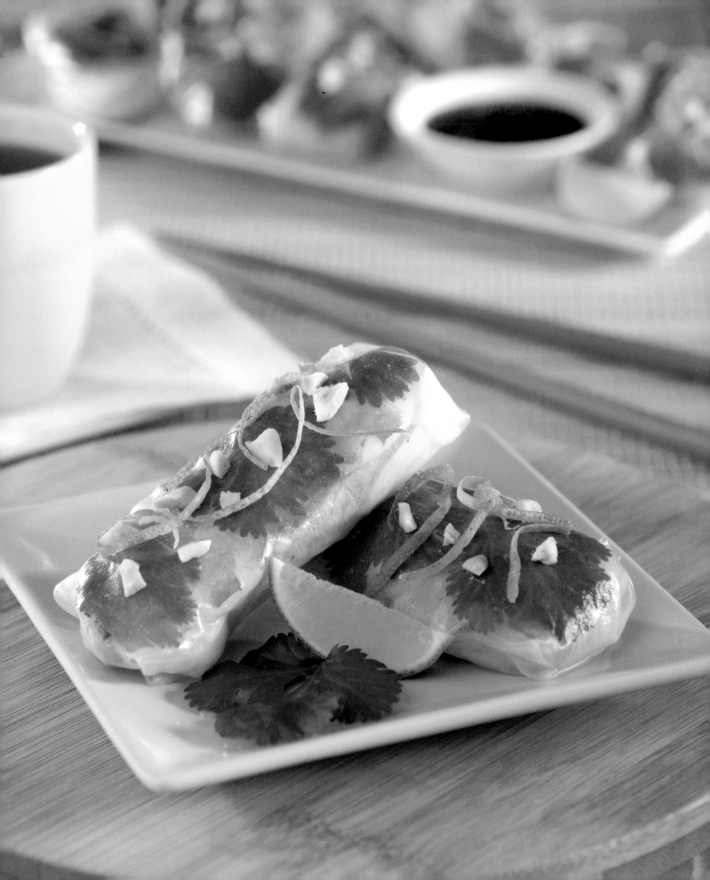

SMOKED SALMON SPREAD

Makes 1½ cups (about 12 servings)

> **8 ounces low-fat cream cheese, softened**
> **3 ounces smoked salmon (lox), coarsely chopped**
> **2 tablespoons fresh lemon juice**
> **1 tablespoon chopped fresh dill, plus additional for garnish**
> **1 tablespoon capers**
> **Cucumber slices, carrot sticks and/or gluten-free crackers**

1. Combine cream cheese, salmon, lemon juice, 1 tablespoon dill and capers in small bowl; mix well.

2. Serve immediately or cover and refrigerate up to 24 hours. Serve with cucumber slices, carrot sticks and/or gluten-free crackers. Garnish with additional dill.

TIP

This savory spread is great for breakfast, too. It can be prepared up to 3 days in advance, covered with plastic wrap and refrigerated.

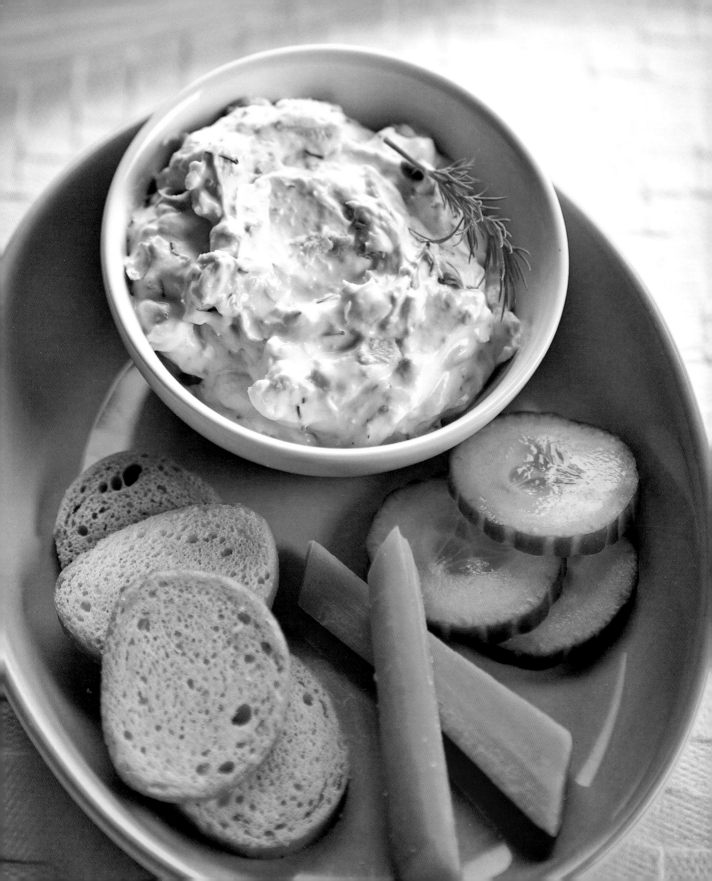

Lunches & Light Meals

QUINOA AND SHRIMP SALAD

Makes 4 servings

      1 cup uncooked quinoa
      2 cups water
      ½ teaspoon salt, divided
      1 package (16 ounces) frozen cooked small shrimp, thawed and well drained
      1 cup grape or cherry tomatoes, halved
      ¼ cup chopped fresh basil
      2 tablespoons capers
      2 tablespoons finely chopped green onion
      3 tablespoons olive oil
      1 to 2 tablespoons lemon juice
      1 teaspoon grated lemon peel
      ⅛ teaspoon black pepper

1. Place quinoa in fine-mesh strainer. Rinse well under cold running water. Bring 2 cups water and ¼ teaspoon salt to a boil in medium saucepan over high heat. Stir in quinoa. Reduce heat to low; cover and simmer 10 to 15 minutes or until quinoa is tender and water is absorbed.

2. Combine quinoa, shrimp, tomatoes, basil, capers and green onion in large bowl. Whisk oil, lemon juice, lemon peel, pepper and remaining ¼ teaspoon salt in small bowl until well blended. Pour over salad; gently toss.

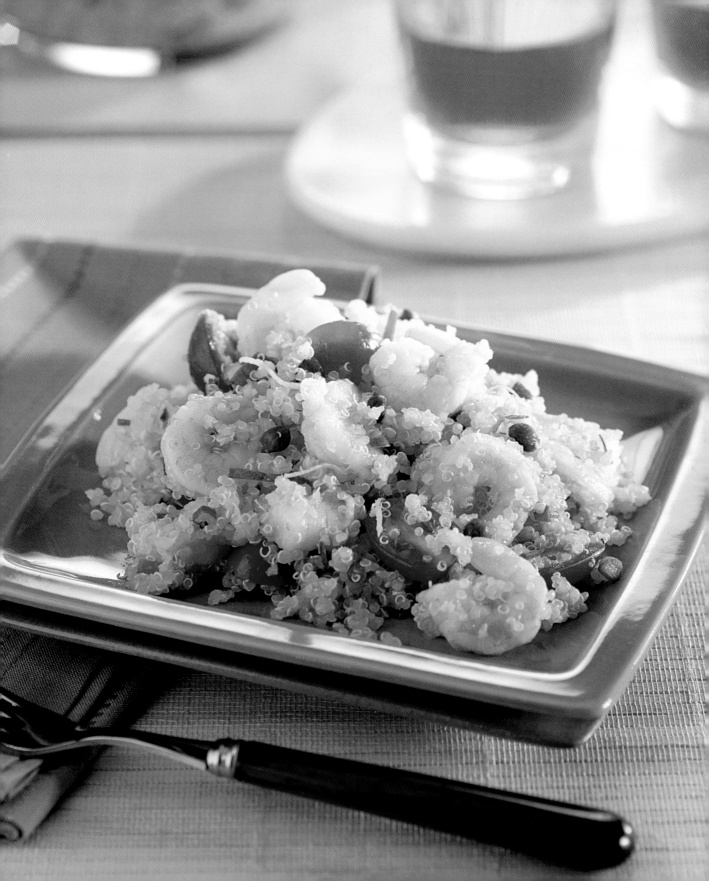

GREEK CHICKEN BURGERS WITH CUCUMBER-YOGURT SAUCE

Makes 4 servings

½ cup plus 2 tablespoons plain nonfat Greek yogurt
½ medium cucumber, peeled, seeded and finely chopped
   Juice of ½ lemon
3 cloves garlic, minced, divided
2 teaspoons finely chopped fresh mint *or* ½ teaspoon dried mint
⅛ teaspoon salt
⅛ teaspoon ground white pepper
1 pound ground chicken breast
3 ounces crumbled feta cheese
4 large kalamata olives, minced
1 egg, lightly beaten
½ teaspoon dried oregano
¼ teaspoon black pepper
   Mixed baby greens and/or fresh mint leaves (optional)

1. Combine yogurt, cucumber, lemon juice, 2 cloves garlic, 2 teaspoons mint, salt and white pepper in medium bowl; mix well. Cover and refrigerate until ready to serve.

2. Combine chicken, cheese, egg, olives, oregano, black pepper and remaining 1 clove garlic in large bowl; mix well. Shape mixture into four patties.

3. Spray grill pan with nonstick cooking spray; heat over medium-high heat. Grill patties 5 to 7 minutes per side or until cooked through (165°F).

4. Serve burgers with sauce and mixed greens, if desired. Garnish with mint leaves.

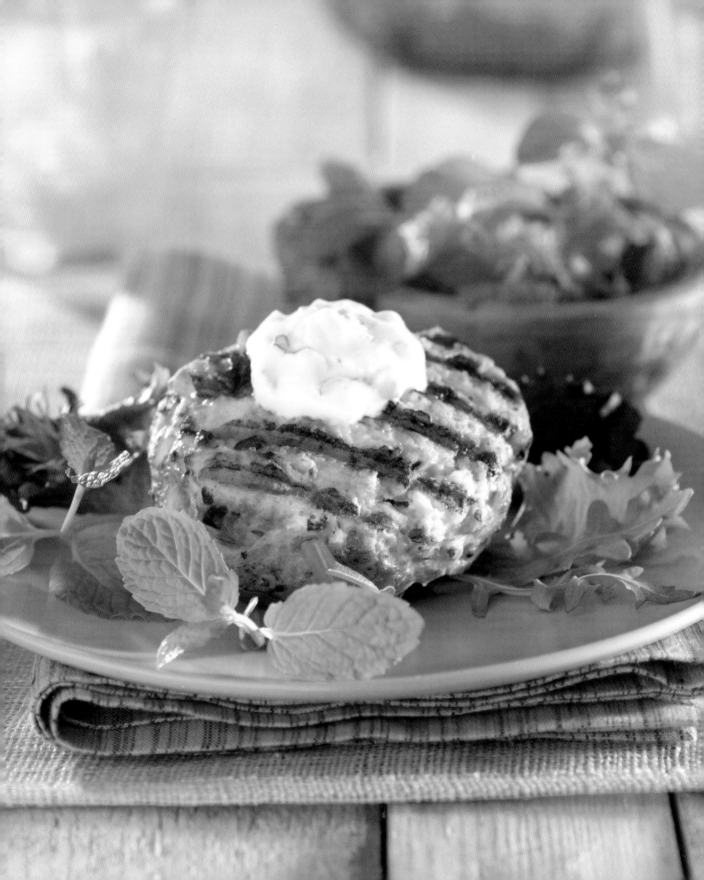

LENTIL VEGETABLE STEW

Makes 8 servings

>   3 tablespoons vegetable oil
>   1 tablespoon curry powder
>   1 tablespoon ground cumin
>   2 teaspoons ground coriander
>   1 teaspoon ground ginger
>   1 large onion, coarsely chopped
> 1½ teaspoons salt
>   1 can (28 ounces) crushed tomatoes
>   2 cups water
>   2 tablespoons cider vinegar
>   2 cups cauliflower florets
>   1 cup chopped red bell pepper
>   1 cup chopped yellow squash
>   1 can (about 15 ounces) lentils, drained

1. Heat oil in large saucepan over medium heat. Add curry powder, cumin, coriander and ginger; cook and stir 1 minute. Add onion and salt, stirring to coat evenly with spice mixture. Cook and stir 5 to 7 minutes or until crisp-tender.

2. Add tomatoes, water and vinegar to saucepan; bring to a simmer. Add cauliflower and bell pepper; reduce heat to medium-low. Simmer 10 minutes.

3. Add squash to saucepan; simmer 20 to 25 minutes or until vegetables are tender. Stir in lentils; cook until heated through.

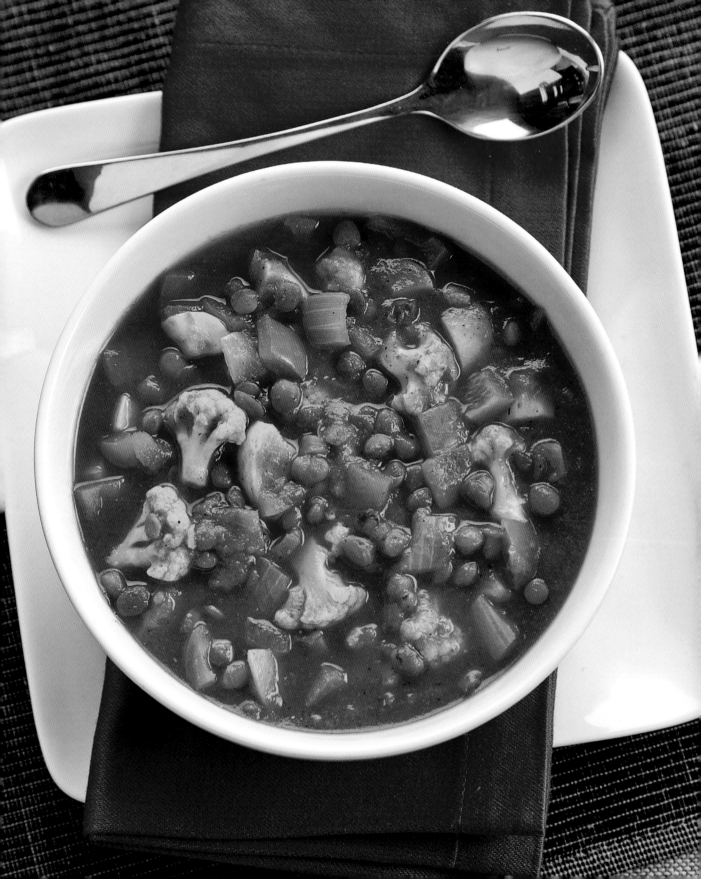

CHICKEN APPLE SALAD

Makes 4 servings

    ¼ cup mayonnaise
    2 tablespoons sour cream
    1 canned chipotle chili pepper in adobo sauce, minced
    ½ teaspoon ground cumin
    ¼ teaspoon salt
    ¼ teaspoon black pepper
    2 cups chopped cooked chicken breast
    1 cup diced unpeeled red or green apple
    ½ cup chopped red bell pepper or roasted red peppers
    ½ cup diced celery
    ⅓ cup raisins
    ⅓ cup diced red onion
  1½ ounces pecan pieces, toasted

1. Stir mayonnaise, sour cream, chipotle pepper, cumin, salt and black pepper in medium bowl until smooth and well blended.

2. Add chicken, apple, bell pepper, celery, raisins and red onion; toss to coat. Stir in pecans just before serving.

TIP

This is a great recipe to take along for a picnic. Enjoy it over lettuce, wrapped in a corn tortilla or in a sandwich.

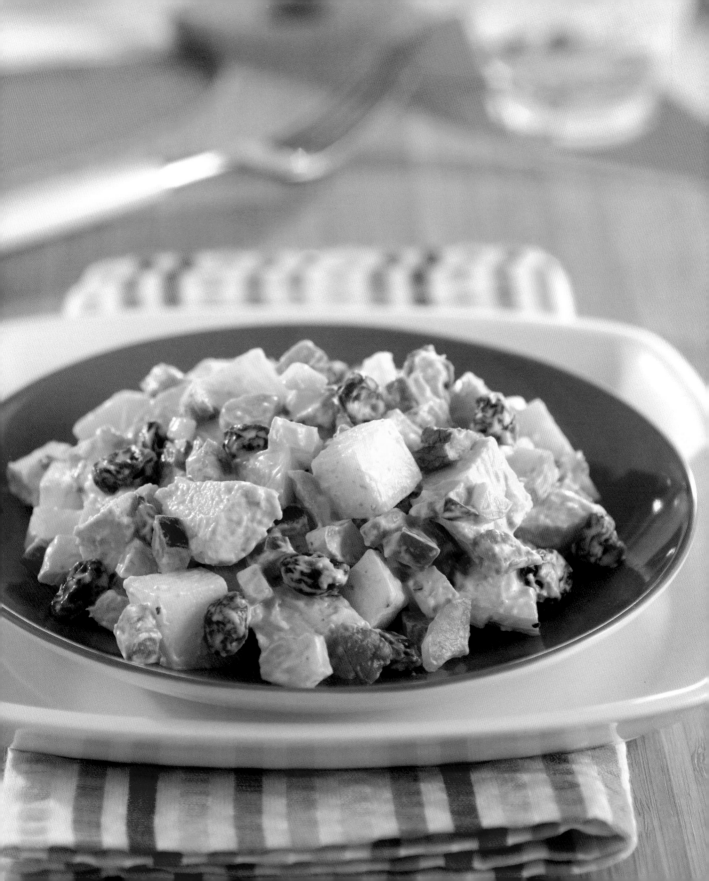

CHICKEN PESTO PIZZAS WITH SPINACH AND TOMATOES

Makes 2 pizzas (about 12 servings)

> 1 package (10.6 ounces) prepared gluten-free pizza crusts
> ⅓ cup pesto sauce
> 1 cup shredded or chopped cooked chicken
> 1 plum tomato, thinly sliced
> ½ cup baby spinach, coarsely chopped
> ⅔ cup shredded part-skim mozzarella cheese

1. Preheat oven to 375°F.

2. Place crusts on pizza pans or baking sheets. Spread pesto evenly over crusts; layer evenly with chicken, tomatoes, spinach and cheese.

3. Bake 12 to 14 minutes or until cheese is melted and crusts are golden brown.

SHRIMP AND AVOCADO TOSTADAS

Makes 4 servings

> 1 cup canned refried black beans
> 8 ounces medium raw shrimp, peeled and deveined
> 3 cloves garlic, minced
> 3 green onions, sliced
> ½ cup salsa
> 1 ripe avocado, diced
> 4 tostada shells, warmed
> ½ cup shredded romaine lettuce
> ½ cup diced tomato

1. Heat small saucepan over medium heat; add refried beans and cook until heated through.

2. Meanwhile, spray large nonstick skillet with nonstick cooking spray; heat over medium-high heat. Add shrimp and garlic; cook and stir 3 minutes or until shrimp are pink and opaque. Add green onions; cook and stir 30 seconds. Stir in salsa; cook until heated through. Remove from heat; gently stir in avocado.

3. Spread beans evenly over tostada shells; top with shrimp mixture, lettuce and tomato.

Chicken Pesto Pizzas with Spinach and Tomatoes

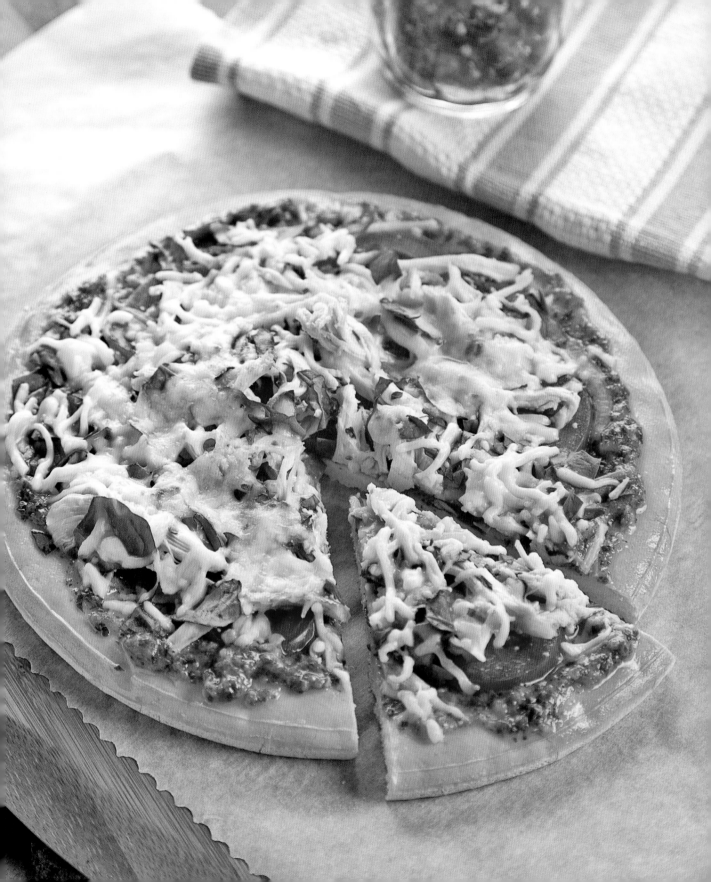

RICE NOODLES WITH BROCCOLI AND TOFU

Makes 4 to 6 servings

> 1 package (14 ounces) firm or extra firm tofu
> 1 package (8 to 10 ounces) wide rice noodles
> 2 tablespoons peanut oil
> 3 medium shallots, sliced
> 6 cloves garlic, minced
> 1 jalapeño pepper,* minced
> 2 teaspoons minced fresh ginger
> 3 cups broccoli florets
> ¼ cup gluten-free soy sauce
> 1 to 2 tablespoons gluten-free fish sauce
> Fresh basil leaves (optional)

Jalapeño peppers can sting and irritate the skin, so wear rubber gloves when handling peppers and do not touch your eyes.

1. Drain tofu and press between paper towels to remove excess water. Cut tofu into bite-size pieces.

2. Meanwhile, place noodles in medium bowl. Cover with hot water; let stand 15 minutes or until tender. Drain.

3. Heat oil in large skillet or wok over medium-high heat. Add tofu; stir-fry 5 minutes or until tofu is lightly browned on all sides. Remove from skillet.

4. Add shallots, garlic, jalapeño and ginger to skillet; stir-fry 2 to 3 minutes. Add broccoli; stir-fry 1 minute. Cover and cook 3 minutes or until broccoli is crisp-tender.

5. Add tofu, noodles, soy sauce and fish sauce to skillet; stir-fry 8 minutes or until heated through. Garnish with basil.

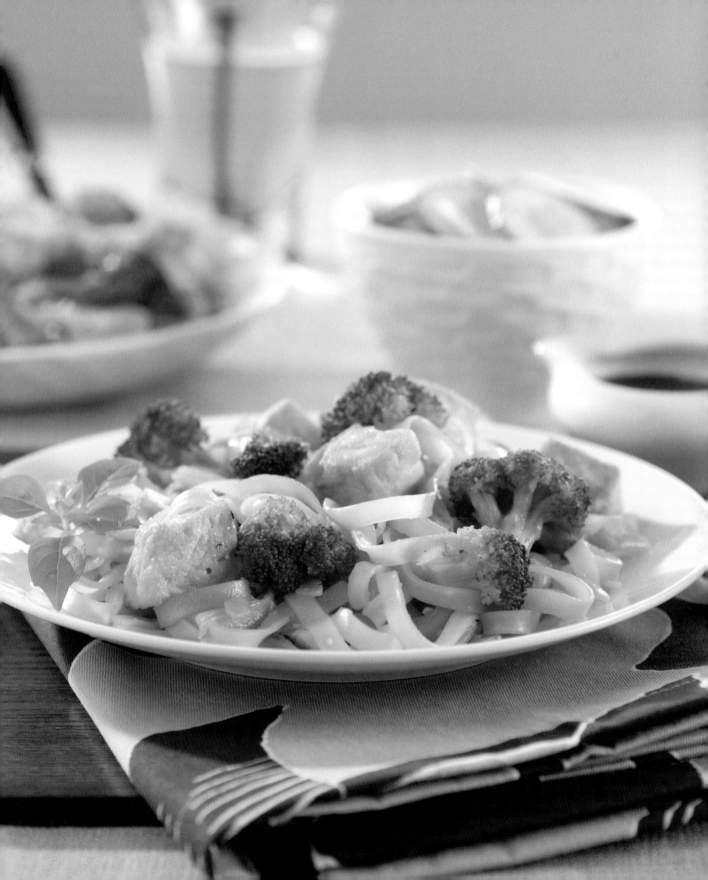

SOUTH-OF-THE-BORDER LUNCH EXPRESS

Makes 2 servings

½ cup chopped seeded tomato

¼ cup chunky salsa

¼ cup rinsed and drained canned black beans

¼ cup frozen corn, thawed

1 teaspoon chopped fresh cilantro

¼ teaspoon chopped garlic

⅛ teaspoon ground red pepper

1 cup cooked brown rice

¼ cup (1 ounce) shredded Cheddar cheese

Microwave Directions

1. Combine tomato, salsa, beans, corn, cilantro, garlic and ground red pepper in 1-quart microwavable bowl. Cover with vented plastic wrap. Microwave on HIGH 1 to 1½ minutes or until heated through; stir.

2. Microwave rice in separate 1-quart microwavable dish on HIGH 1 to 1½ minutes or until heated through. Top with tomato mixture and cheese.

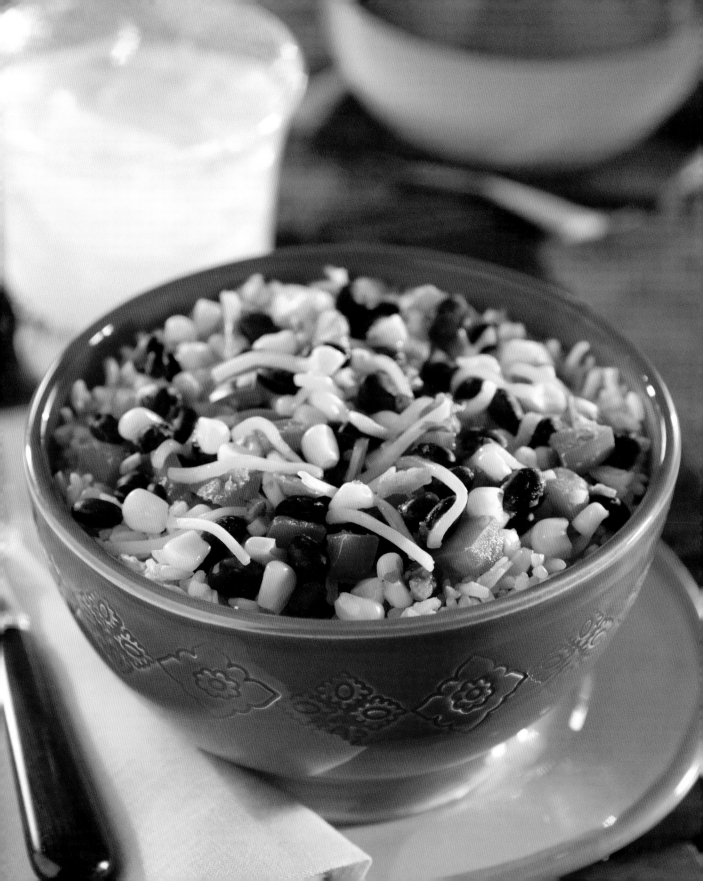

TURKEY LETTUCE WRAPS

Makes 12 wraps (about 6 servings)

  1 teaspoon sesame oil
  1 pound ground turkey
 ½ cup sliced green onions
  2 tablespoons minced fresh ginger
  1 can (8 ounces) water chestnuts, chopped
  1 teaspoon gluten-free soy sauce
 ¼ cup chopped fresh cilantro
 12 large lettuce leaves
    Chopped mint leaves and/or chopped peanuts (optional)

1. Heat oil in large skillet over medium-high heat. Add turkey, green onions and ginger; cook 6 to 8 minutes, stirring to break up meat.

2. Add water chestnuts and soy sauce to skillet; cook 3 minutes or until turkey is no longer pink. Remove from heat; stir in cilantro.

3. Spoon ¼ cup turkey mixture into each lettuce leaf. Top with chopped mint and and/or peanuts, if desired. Roll up to enclose filling.

Variations: Use turkey mixture as a salad topping or substitute corn tortillas for the lettuce leaves.

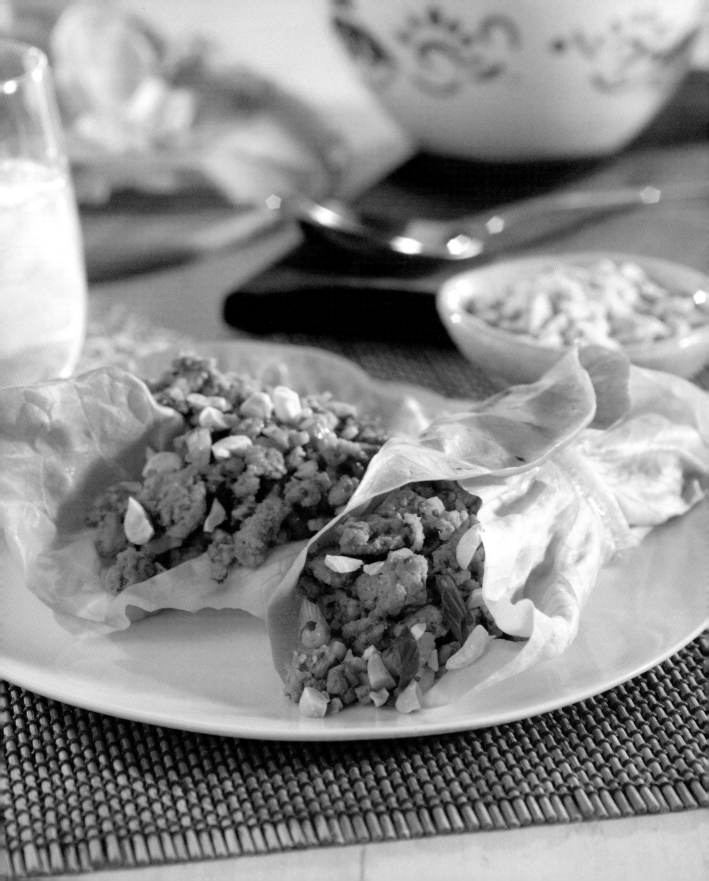

STUFFED SQUASH WITH BLACK BEANS

Makes 4 servings

 1 cup water, divided
 1 acorn squash (2 pounds), quartered, seeded, skin pierced with fork
   Salt and black pepper
 ⅓ cup pine nuts (1½ ounces)
 1 cup chopped onion
 1 medium red bell pepper, chopped
 1 teaspoon ground cinnamon
 ¼ teaspoon ground allspice (optional)
 1 cup canned black beans, rinsed and drained
 ¼ cup raisins
 1 teaspoon sugar
 ¼ teaspoon salt
 2 ounces crumbled goat or feta cheese

1. Pour ½ cup water into large microwavable dish. Place squash, skin side up, in dish. Sprinkle with salt and black pepper. Cover with plastic wrap. Microwave on HIGH 12 minutes or until tender.

2. Meanwhile, heat medium nonstick skillet over medium-high heat. Add pine nuts; cook and stir 1 minute or until lightly browned. Remove to plate.

3. Spray skillet with nonstick cooking spray. Add onion and bell pepper; cook and stir 5 minutes or until vegetables just begin to brown. Add cinnamon and allspice, if desired; cook and stir 30 seconds. Add beans, raisins, sugar and ¼ teaspoon salt. Stir in remaining ½ cup water. Remove from heat. Cover; let stand 2 minutes.

4. Place squash pieces on four serving plates. Spoon bean mixture into center of each squash piece. Sprinkle with pine nuts and cheese.

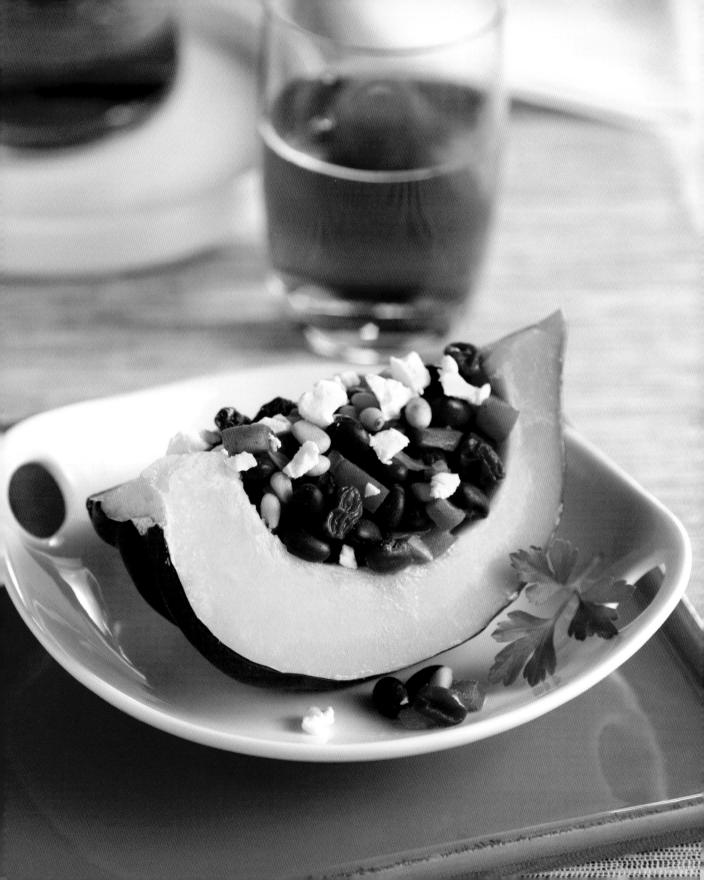

CAJUN SAUSAGE GRITS

Makes 4 servings

2¼ cups water
½ cup quick-cooking grits
2 teaspoons canola oil
6 ounces Cajun-style andouille chicken sausage, thinly sliced
1 cup diced green bell pepper
1 cup diced onion
½ teaspoon dried thyme
1 cup grape tomatoes, halved
¼ cup chopped fresh parsley
4 teaspoons gluten-free hot pepper sauce

1. Bring water to a boil in medium saucepan over high heat. Gradually stir in grits; reduce heat. Cover and simmer 6 minutes or until thickened, stirring occasionally. Set aside.

2. Meanwhile, heat oil in large nonstick skillet over medium-high heat. Add sausage; cook and stir 3 minutes. Add bell pepper, onion and thyme; cook and stir 4 minutes or until lightly browned. Stir in tomatoes; cook 2 minutes or until just beginning to soften. Remove from heat.

3. Stir parsley and hot pepper sauce into skillet. Cover and let stand 5 minutes to allow flavors to blend. Serve over grits.

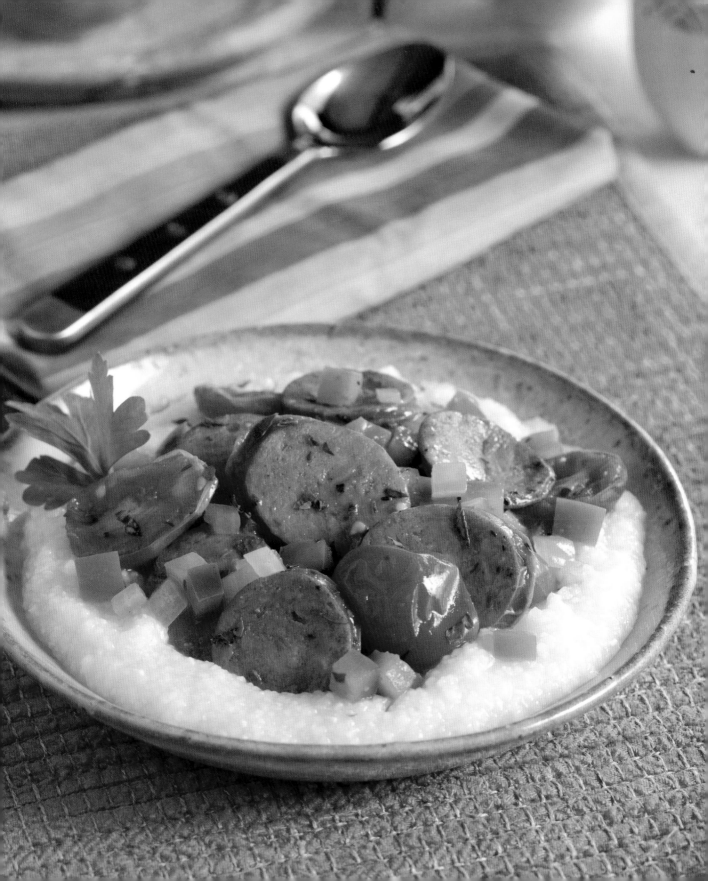

CURRIED CHICKEN WRAPS

Makes 4 wraps (about 2 servings)

⅓ cup mayonnaise
2 tablespoons mango chutney
½ teaspoon curry powder
4 (6-inch) corn tortillas
1½ cups shredded coleslaw mix
1½ cups shredded or chopped cooked chicken
2 tablespoons chopped lightly salted peanuts
1 tablespoon chopped fresh cilantro, plus additional for garnish

1. Combine mayonnaise, chutney and curry powder in small bowl; mix well. Spread evenly onto one side of each tortilla.

2. Top evenly with coleslaw mix, chicken, peanuts and 1 tablespoon cilantro. Roll up to enclose filling. Cut in half diagonally to serve. Garnish with additional cilantro.

GRILLED FISH TACOS

Makes 8 tacos (about 4 servings)

¾ teaspoon chili powder
1 pound skinless mahimahi, halibut or tilapia fillets
½ cup salsa, divided
2 cups shredded coleslaw mix or cabbage
¼ cup sour cream
4 tablespoons chopped fresh cilantro, divided
8 (6-inch) corn tortillas, warmed

1. Prepare grill for direct cooking. Sprinkle chili powder evenly over fish. Spoon ¼ cup salsa over fish; let stand 10 minutes.

2. Meanwhile, combine coleslaw mix, remaining ¼ cup salsa, sour cream and 2 tablespoons cilantro in large bowl; mix well.

3. Grill fish, salsa side up, covered, over medium heat 8 to 10 minutes or until fish is opaque in center and begins to flake when tested with fork.

4. Slice fish crosswise into thin strips or cut into chunks. Fill warm tortillas with fish and coleslaw mix. Garnish with remaining 2 tablespoons cilantro.

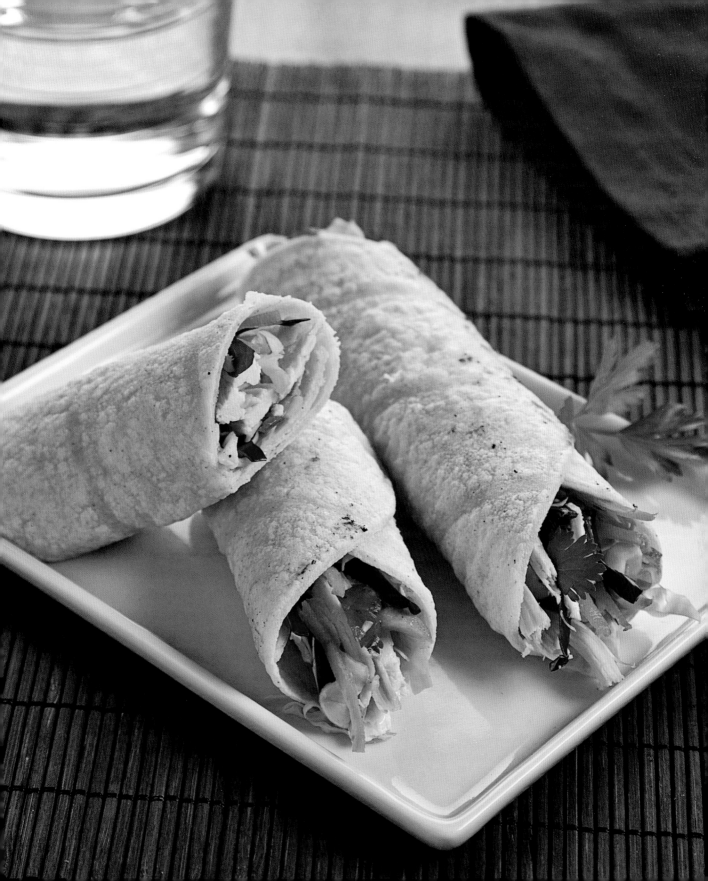

SPAGHETTI SQUASH PRIMAVERA

Makes 4 servings

    1 spaghetti squash (about 2 pounds)
    2 teaspoons canola oil
    ½ teaspoon finely chopped garlic
    ¼ cup finely chopped red onion
    ¼ cup thinly sliced carrot
    ¼ cup thinly sliced red bell pepper
    ¼ cup thinly sliced green bell pepper
    1 can (about 14 ounces) Italian-style stewed tomatoes
    ½ cup thinly sliced yellow squash
    ½ cup thinly sliced zucchini
    ½ cup frozen corn, thawed
    ½ teaspoon dried oregano
    ⅛ teaspoon dried thyme
    4 teaspoons grated Parmesan cheese
    2 tablespoons finely chopped fresh parsley

1. Cut spaghetti squash lengthwise in half; remove seeds. Place squash, cut side down, in large microwavable dish. Cover with vented plastic wrap. Microwave on HIGH 9 minutes or until squash separates easily into strands when tested with fork.

2. Meanwhile, heat oil in large skillet over medium heat. Add garlic; cook and stir 1 minute. Add onion, carrot and bell peppers; cook and stir 3 minutes. Add tomatoes, yellow squash, zucchini, corn, oregano and thyme; bring to a boil. Reduce heat; simmer 5 minutes or until vegetables are tender, stirring occasionally.

3. Separate squash strands with fork. Spoon vegetables evenly over squash. Top with cheese and parsley just before serving.

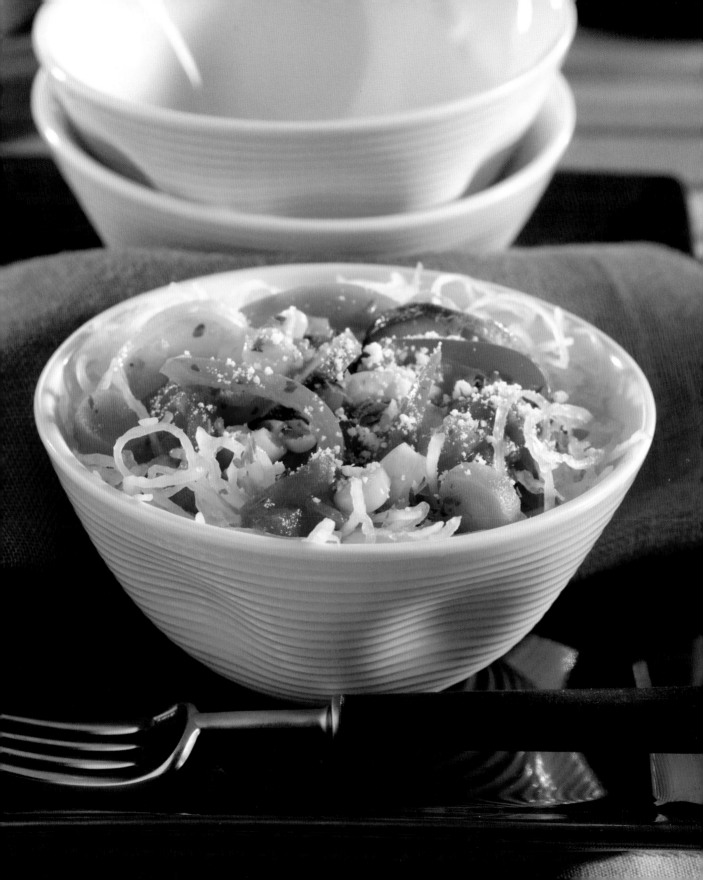

TORTILLA PIZZA WEDGES

Makes 4 servings

1 cup frozen corn, thawed
1 cup thinly sliced fresh mushrooms
4 (6-inch) corn tortillas
¼ cup gluten-free pasta sauce
1 to 2 teaspoons chopped jalapeño pepper*
¼ teaspoon dried oregano
¼ teaspoon dried marjoram
½ cup (2 ounces) shredded mozzarella cheese

Jalapeño peppers can sting and irritate the skin, so wear rubber gloves when handling peppers and do not touch your eyes.

1. Preheat oven to 450°F. Spray large skillet with cooking spray; heat over medium heat. Add corn and mushrooms; cook and stir 4 to 5 minutes or until tender.

2. Place tortillas on baking sheet. Bake 4 minutes or until edges begin to brown.

3. Combine pasta sauce, jalapeño, oregano and marjoram in small bowl. Spread evenly over tortillas. Top evenly with corn and mushrooms. Sprinkle with cheese.

4. Bake 4 to 5 minutes or until cheese is melted and pizzas are heated through. Cut each pizza into four wedges.

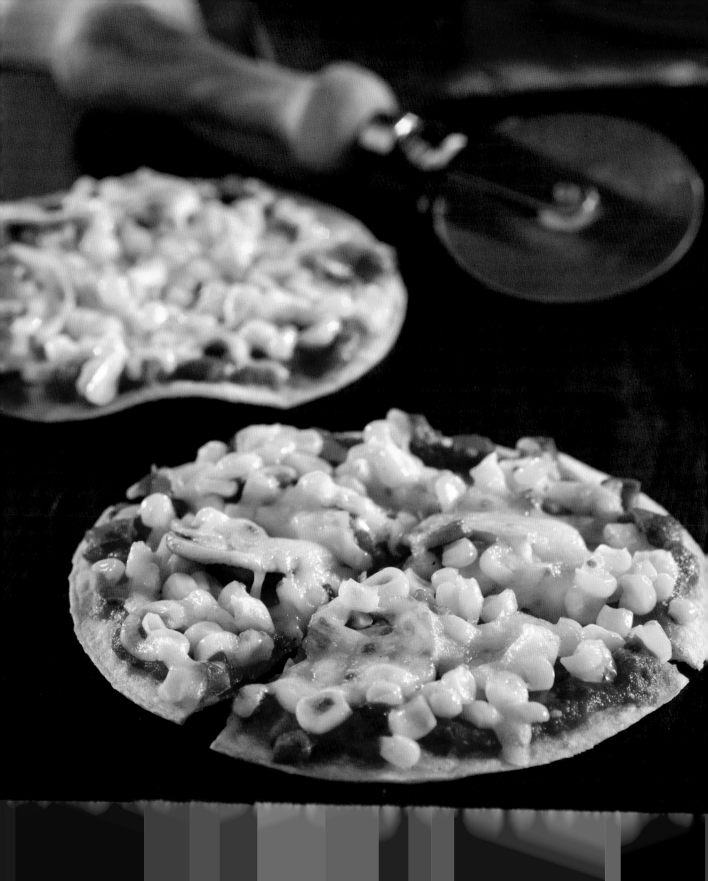

TUNA SALAD STUFFED SWEET RED PEPPERS

Makes 4 servings

> **2 cans (5 ounces each) albacore tuna in water, drained and flaked**
> **2 stalks celery, sliced diagonally**
> **½ cup halved green grapes**
> **½ cup (2 ounces) shredded sharp Cheddar cheese**
> **⅓ cup mayonnaise**
>   **Salt and black pepper**
> **2 red bell peppers, halved and seeded**

1. Combine tuna, celery, grapes, cheese and mayonnaise in medium bowl; mix well. Season with salt and black pepper.

2. Divide tuna mixture evenly among hollowed bell pepper halves.

TIP

This makes a great portable lunch for school or the office. Pack the tuna salad into a reusable plastic food storage container. Pack the bell peppers in a resealable food storage bag. Refrigerate until ready to serve. To assemble for lunch, spoon the tuna salad into the bell pepper halves.

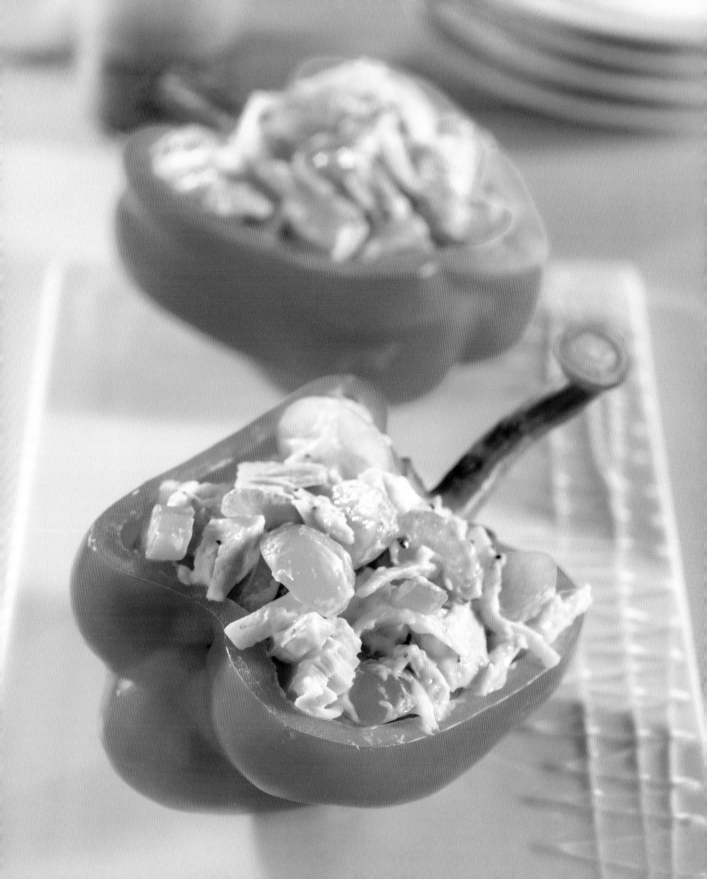

Everyday Dinners

APPLE-CHERRY GLAZED PORK CHOPS

Makes 2 servings

- ¼ to ½ teaspoon dried thyme
- ⅛ teaspoon salt
- ⅛ teaspoon black pepper
- 2 boneless pork loin chops (3 ounces each), trimmed of fat
- ⅔ cup unsweetened apple juice
- ½ small apple, sliced
- 2 tablespoons sliced green onion
- 2 tablespoons dried tart cherries
- 1 teaspoon cornstarch
- 1 tablespoon water

1. Combine thyme, salt and pepper in small bowl. Rub onto both sides of pork chops.

2. Spray large skillet with cooking spray; heat over medium heat. Add pork chops; cook 3 to 5 minutes or until barely pink in center, turning once. Remove to plate; keep warm.

3. Add apple juice, apple slices, green onion and cherries to same skillet. Simmer 2 to 3 minutes or until apple and onion are tender.

4. Stir cornstarch into water in small bowl until smooth; stir into skillet. Bring to a boil; cook and stir until thickened. Spoon apple mixture over pork chops.

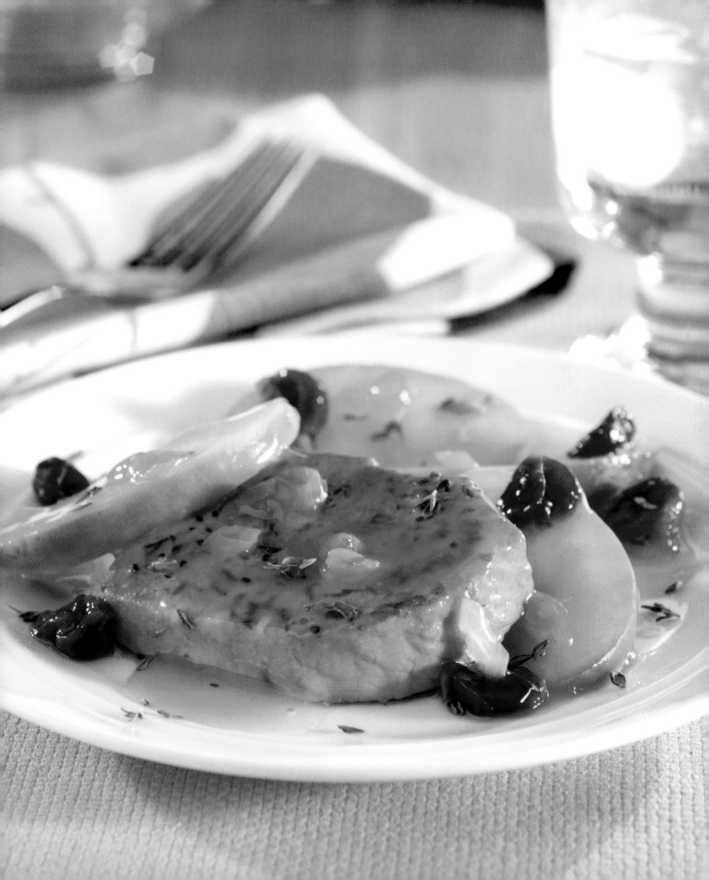

BAKED PENNE WITH SAUSAGE AND PEPPERS

Makes 8 servings

8 ounces gluten-free brown rice penne pasta
1 tablespoon olive oil
1 pound hot or mild Italian sausage, casings removed
1 yellow bell pepper, cut into ½-inch pieces
1 green bell pepper, cut into ½-inch pieces
1 jar (24 ounces) gluten-free spicy tomato-basil marinara sauce
2 cups (8 ounces) shredded mozzarella cheese, divided
   Chopped fresh basil (optional)

1. Preheat oven to 350°F.

2. Cook pasta according to package directions until al dente. Drain; cover and keep warm.

3. Meanwhile, heat oil in large nonstick skillet over medium heat. Crumble sausage into skillet; cook 5 minutes or until browned, stirring to break up meat. Add bell peppers; cook 5 to 7 minutes or until sausage is no longer pink and bell peppers are crisp-tender. Drain fat.

4. Add marinara sauce to skillet; cook 3 minutes or until heated through. Stir in penne.

5. Spread half of penne mixture in 2-quart casserole. Top with 1 cup cheese. Layer with remaining penne mixture and 1 cup cheese.

6. Bake 25 to 30 minutes or until heated through and cheese is melted. Garnish with basil.

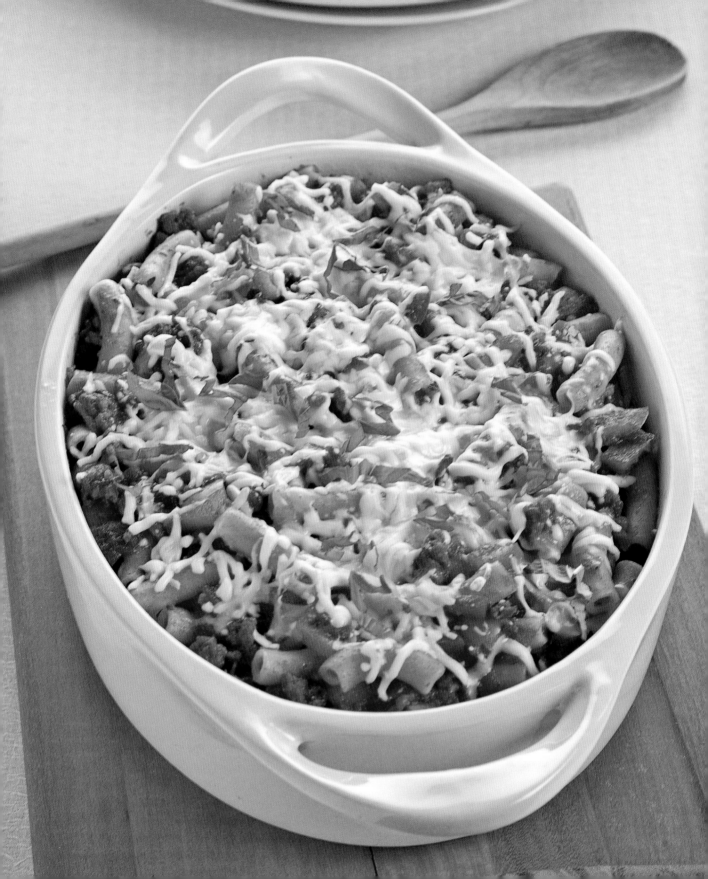

VEGETARIAN PAELLA

Makes 6 servings

   2 teaspoons canola oil
   1 cup chopped onion
   2 cloves garlic, minced
   1 cup brown rice
2¼ cups vegetable broth
   1 can (about 14 ounces) stewed tomatoes
   1 small zucchini, sliced into ½-inch pieces (about 1¼ cups)
   1 cup chopped red bell pepper
   2 teaspoons Italian seasoning
   ½ teaspoon ground turmeric
   ⅛ teaspoon ground red pepper
   1 can (14 ounces) quartered artichoke hearts, drained
   ½ cup frozen baby peas
   ¾ teaspoon salt

Slow Cooker Directions

1. Heat oil in small nonstick skillet over medium-high heat. Add onion; cook and stir 6 to 7 minutes or until tender. Stir in garlic. Transfer to slow cooker. Stir in rice.

2. Add broth, tomatoes, zucchini, bell pepper, Italian seasoning, turmeric and ground red pepper; mix well. Cover; cook on LOW 4 hours or on HIGH 2 hours or until liquid is absorbed.

3. Stir in artichokes, peas and salt. Cover; cook 5 to 10 minutes or until vegetables are tender.

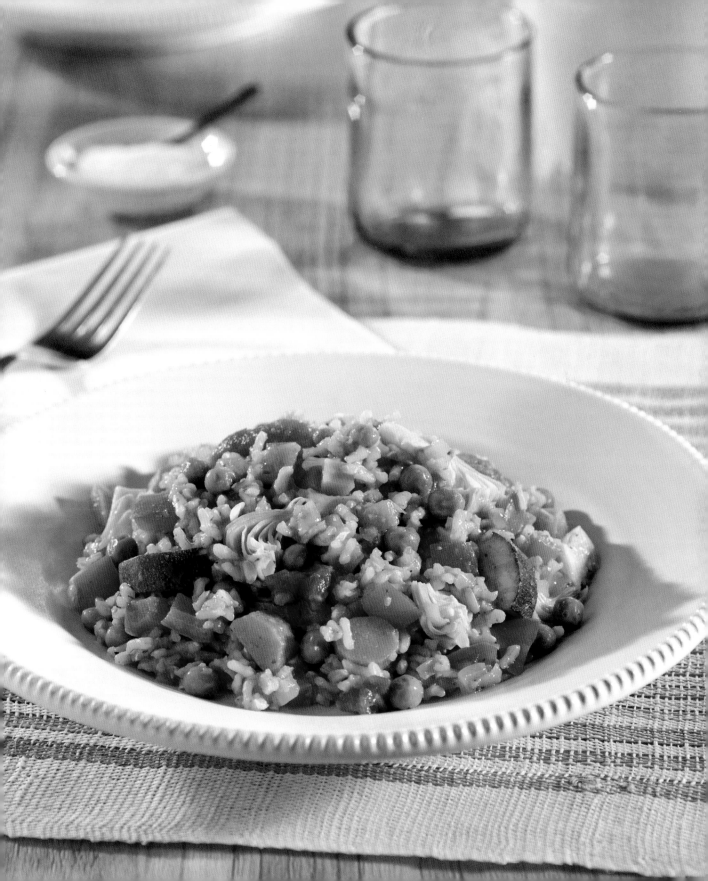

BEEF AND BEAN ENCHILADAS

Makes 4 servings

    8 ounces ground beef
    1 can (about 15 ounces) pinto beans, rinsed and drained
    ½ teaspoon ground cumin
    ½ teaspoon salt, divided
    ¼ teaspoon black pepper, divided
    1 tablespoon canola oil
    1 onion, chopped
    1 green bell pepper, chopped
    1 jalapeño pepper,* minced (optional)
    1 clove garlic, minced
    1 can (about 14 ounces) crushed tomatoes
  1½ teaspoons chili powder
    8 (5-inch) corn tortillas, softened according to package directions

Jalapeño peppers can sting and irritate the skin, so wear rubber gloves when handling peppers and do not touch your eyes.

1. Preheat oven to 350°F. Brown beef in large skillet over medium-high heat 6 to 8 minutes, stirring to break up meat. Drain fat.

2. Mash beans in large bowl. Stir in cumin, ¼ teaspoon salt and ⅛ teaspoon black pepper. Add beef; mix well.

3. Heat oil in same skillet over medium heat. Add onion, bell pepper, jalapeño, if desired, and garlic; cook and stir 8 to 10 minutes or until onion is translucent.

4. Stir tomatoes, chili powder, remaining ¼ teaspoon salt and ⅛ teaspoon black pepper into skillet. Reduce heat to low; simmer 5 minutes.

5. To assemble enchiladas, spoon ¼ cup bean mixture down center of each tortilla. Fold ends to center to enclose filling. Place in 9-inch square baking dish. Top evenly with tomato sauce. Bake 20 minutes or until heated through.

Serving Suggestion: Serve with rice and a fresh green salad.

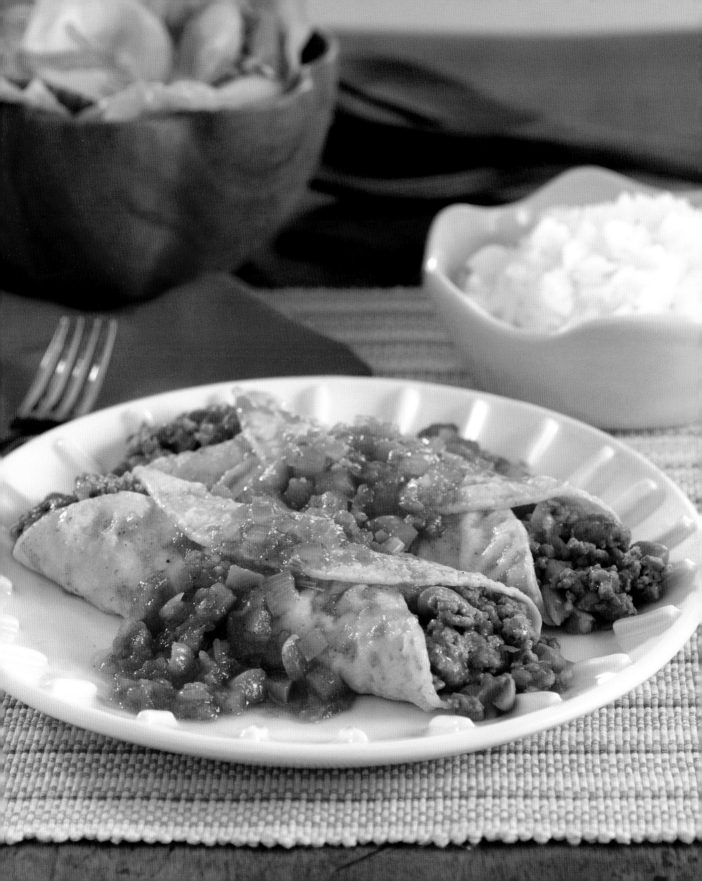

ORANGE CHICKEN STIR-FRY OVER QUINOA

Makes 4 servings

½ cup uncooked quinoa
1 cup water
⅛ teaspoon salt
2 teaspoons vegetable oil, divided
1 pound boneless skinless chicken breasts, cut into thin strips
1 cup fresh squeezed orange juice (2 to 3 oranges)
1 tablespoon gluten-free soy sauce
1 tablespoon cornstarch
½ cup sliced green onion
2 tablespoons grated fresh ginger
6 ounces snow peas, ends trimmed
1 cup thinly sliced carrots
¼ teaspoon red pepper flakes (optional)

1. Place quinoa in fine-mesh strainer; rinse well under cold running water. Bring 1 cup water to a boil in medium saucepan; stir in quinoa. Reduce heat to low; cover and simmer 10 to 15 minutes or until quinoa is tender and water is absorbed. Stir in salt.

2. Meanwhile, heat 1 teaspoon oil in large skillet over medium-high heat. Add chicken; cook and stir 4 to 6 minutes or until no longer pink. Remove to plate; keep warm.

3. Stir orange juice and soy sauce into cornstarch in small bowl until smooth; set aside. Heat remaining 1 teaspoon oil in skillet. Add green onion and ginger; stir-fry 1 to 2 minutes. Add snow peas and carrots; stir-fry 4 to 5 minutes or until carrots are crisp-tender.

4. Return chicken to skillet. Stir orange juice mixture; add to skillet. Bring to a boil. Reduce heat; simmer until slightly thickened.

5. Serve chicken and vegetables over quinoa; sprinkle with red pepper flakes, if desired.

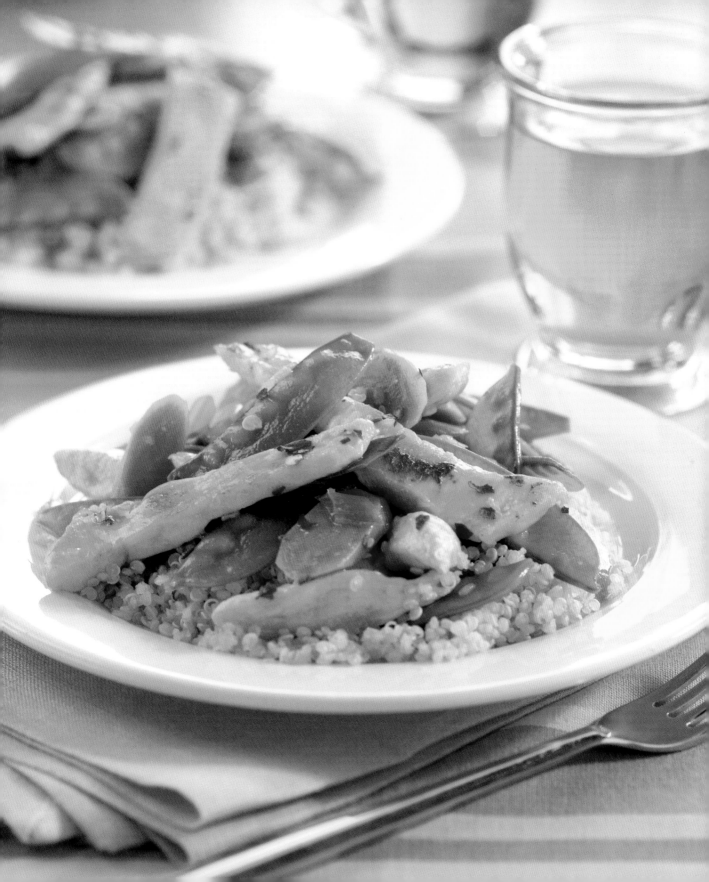

BUTTERNUT SQUASH GNOCCHI WITH SAVORY HERB BUTTER

Makes 4 servings

1 butternut squash (about 2½ pounds), peeled, seeded and cut into 1-inch pieces
1 cup rice flour, plus additional for work surface
3½ teaspoons salt, divided
1 teaspoon xanthan gum
¼ teaspoon black pepper
4 quarts water
¼ cup (½ stick) butter
2 teaspoons minced garlic
1 teaspoon dried parsley
1 teaspoon rubbed sage
½ teaspoon dried thyme
Juice of 1 lemon
¼ cup shredded Parmesan cheese

1. Place squash in large microwavable bowl. Cover with vented plastic wrap. Microwave on HIGH 6 to 7 minutes or until very tender. Let stand 10 minutes to cool slightly. Drain.

2. Mash squash or press through ricer into medium bowl. Add 1 cup rice flour, 2 teaspoons salt, xanthan gum and pepper; mix well.

3. Heavily dust cutting board or work surface with rice flour. Working in batches, scoop portions of dough onto board and roll into ½-inch-thick rope using rice-floured hands. Cut each rope into ¾-inch pieces.

4. Bring water and 1 teaspoon salt to a boil in large saucepan over high heat. Drop 8 to 12 gnocchi into boiling water; cook about 2½ minutes or until gnocchi float to surface. Remove gnocchi with slotted spoon; drain on paper towels. Return water to a boil; repeat with remaining gnocchi.

5. Combine butter, garlic, parsley, sage, thyme and remaining ½ teaspoon salt in large nonstick skillet. Heat over medium heat until butter is melted and just begins to brown. Add lemon juice; cook 30 seconds. Add gnocchi; gently toss to coat. Cook 2 minutes or until lightly browned and heated through.

6. Divide gnocchi among four serving bowls. Top with cheese.

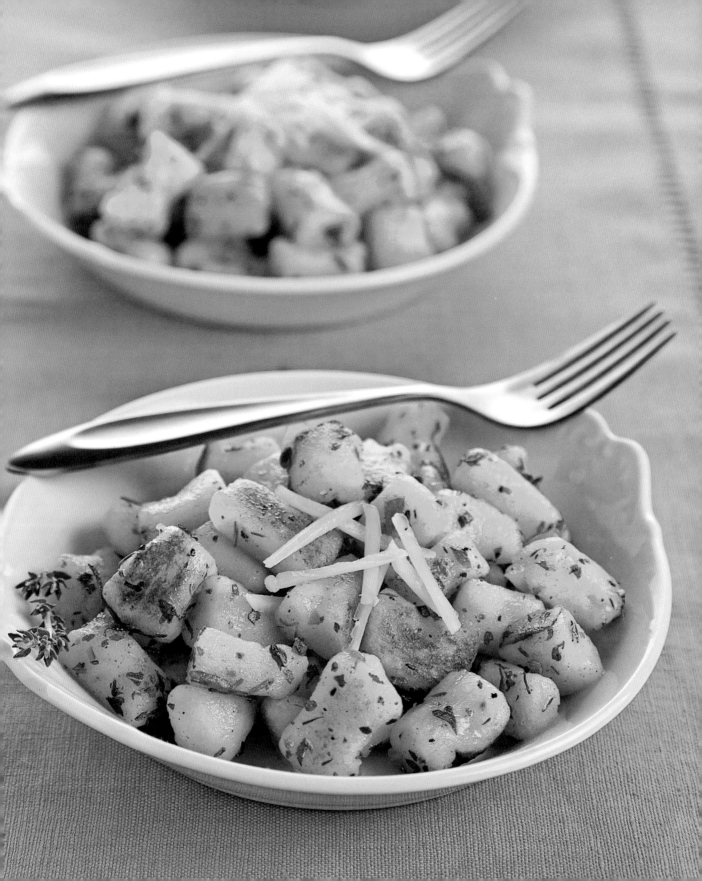

PECAN CATFISH WITH CRANBERRY COMPOTE

Makes 4 servings

    Cranberry Compote (recipe follows)
2 **tablespoons butter, divided**
1½ **cups pecans**
2 **tablespoons rice flour**
1 **egg**
2 **tablespoons water**
    Salt and black pepper
4 **catfish fillets (about 1¼ pounds)**

1. Preheat oven to 425°F. Prepare Cranberry Compote; set aside.

2. Melt 1 tablespoon butter; place in 13×9-inch baking pan, tilting pan to coat evenly Combine pecans and rice flour in food processor; pulse just until finely chopped.

3. Place pecan mixture in shallow dish. Whisk egg and water in another shallow dish. Season both sides of each fillet with salt and pepper. Dip fillets in egg mixture, letting excess drip back into dish. Coat fish in pecan mixture, pressing to lightly to adhere. Place in prepared pan. Dot with remaining 1 tablespoon butter.

4. Bake 15 to 20 minutes or until fish begins to flake when tested with fork. Serve with Cranberry Compote.

CRANBERRY COMPOTE

Makes about 3 cups

    1 **package (12 ounces) fresh cranberries**
¾ **cup water**
⅔ **cup sugar**
¼ **cup orange juice**
2 **teaspoons grated fresh ginger**
¼ **teaspoon Chinese five-spice powder**
⅛ **teaspoon salt**
1 **teaspoon butter**

continued on page 148

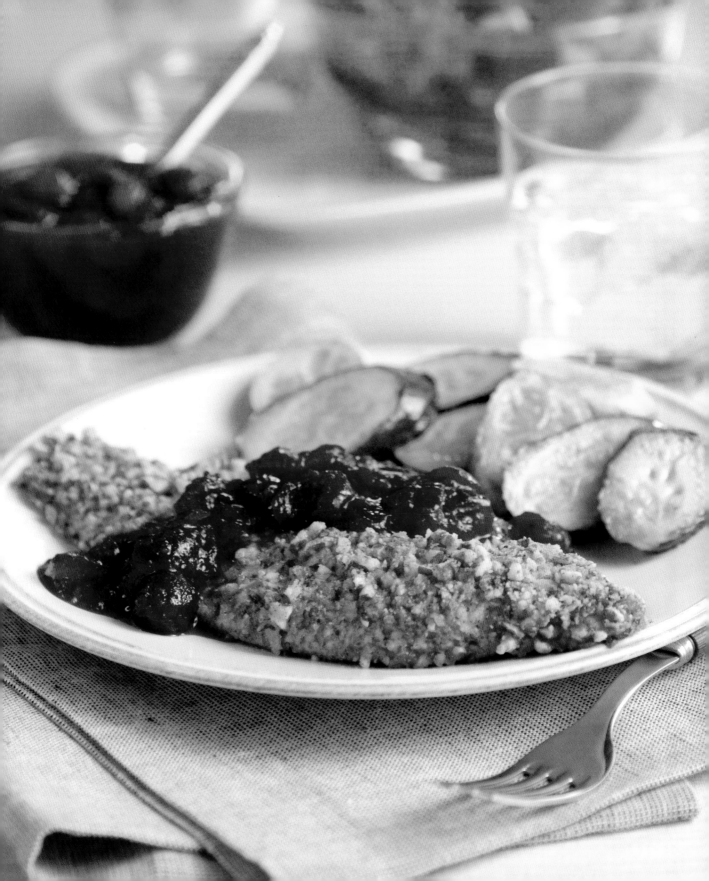

Pecan Catfish with Cranberry Compote, continued

1. Wash and pick over cranberries. Combine cranberries, water, sugar, orange juice, ginger, five-spice powder and salt in large saucepan. Cook over medium-high heat 10 minutes or until berries begin to pop, stirring occasionally. Cook and stir 5 minutes or until sauce is thickened.

2. Remove from heat; stir in butter until melted. Let stand 10 minutes.

NEPTUNE'S SPAGHETTI SQUASH

Makes 4 servings

> 1 spaghetti squash (about 2 pounds)
> 3 tablespoons olive oil
> 1 clove garlic, minced
> 8 ounces medium raw shrimp (with tails on), peeled and deveined
> 8 ounces bay scallops
> ½ cup fresh or frozen peas
> ¼ cup sun-dried tomatoes in oil, drained and chopped
> ½ teaspoon dried basil
> ¼ cup grated Parmesan cheese

1. Cut spaghetti squash in half lengthwise; remove seeds. Place squash, cut side down, in large microwavable dish. Cover with vented plastic wrap. Microwave on HIGH 9 minutes or until squash separates easily into strands when tested with fork.

2. Meanwhile, heat oil in large skillet over medium-high heat. Add garlic; cook and stir 1 minute. Add shrimp, scallops, peas, tomatoes and basil; cook and stir 1 to 2 minutes or until shrimp are pink and opaque and scallops are opaque.

3. Separate squash strands with fork. Divide evenly among four bowls. Top squash with seafood mixture; gently toss. Sprinkle with cheese.

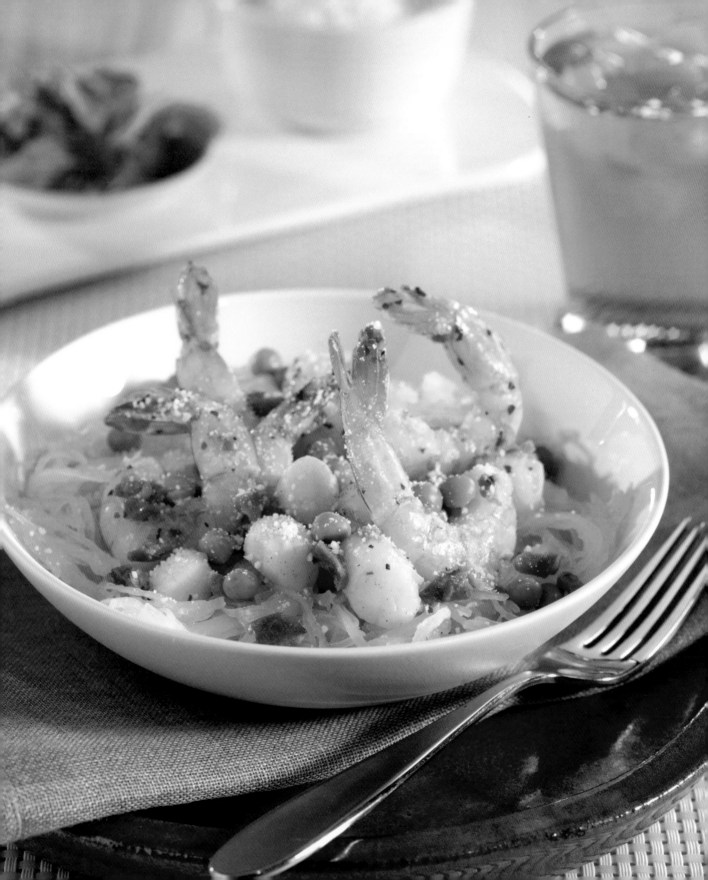

TAMALE PIE

Makes 4 servings

Topping

>   ¾ to 1 cup gluten-free biscuit baking mix
>   ½ cup milk
>   1 egg
>   2 tablespoons butter, melted
>   ½ jalapeño pepper,* finely chopped

Filling

>   1 tablespoon olive oil
>   1 green bell pepper, chopped
>   ¾ cup chopped green onions
>   2 cloves garlic, finely chopped
>   ½ pound ground turkey
>   1½ cups canned crushed tomatoes
>   1 can (about 15 ounces) pinto beans, rinsed and drained
>   2 teaspoons chili powder
>   1 teaspoon ground cumin
>   ¼ teaspoon black pepper

Jalapeño peppers can sting and irritate the skin, so wear rubber gloves when handling peppers and do not touch your eyes.

1. Preheat oven to 425°F. Spray 9-inch pie plate with nonstick cooking spray.

2. For topping, stir baking mix, milk, egg, butter and jalapeño in medium bowl until well blended;** set aside.

3. For filling, heat oil in large nonstick skillet over medium heat. Add bell pepper, green onions and garlic; cook and stir 5 minutes or until vegetables are tender. Add turkey; cook and stir until no longer pink. Add tomatoes, beans, chili powder, cumin and black pepper; cook and stir 5 minutes or until heated through.

4. Spoon vegetable mixture into prepared pie plate. Drop heaping tablespoonfuls of topping over filling.

5. Bake 25 to 30 minutes or until topping is golden brown. Let stand 5 minutes before serving.

**The consistency of the topping will vary depending on the baking mix used in the recipe. Be sure the batter is smooth and thick. If is too thin, it will spread.*

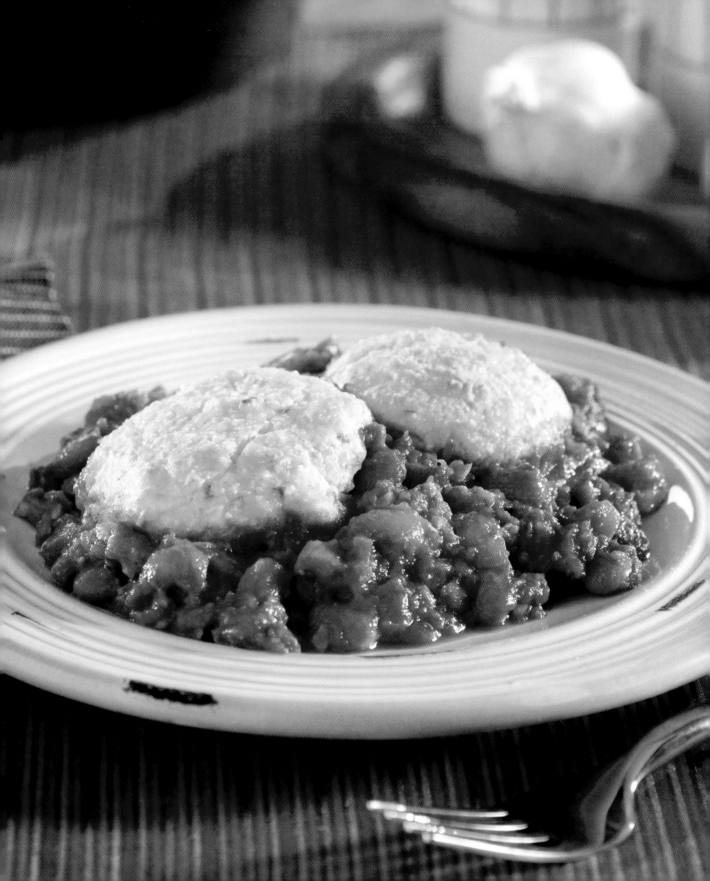

CHICKEN AND VEGETABLE RISOTTO

Makes 4 servings

6 cups gluten-free chicken broth
2 tablespoons olive oil
2 cups sliced mushrooms
½ cup chopped onion
4 cloves garlic, minced
1½ cups uncooked arborio rice
1 pound cooked chicken tenders, cut into 1½-inch pieces
2 cups cooked broccoli florets
4 plum tomatoes, seeded and chopped
¼ cup finely chopped fresh parsley *or* 1 tablespoon dried parsley flakes
3 to 4 tablespoons finely chopped fresh basil *or* 1 tablespoon dried basil
½ teaspoon salt
½ teaspoon black pepper
2 tablespoons grated Parmesan or Romano cheese

1. Bring broth to a boil in medium saucepan; reduce heat to a simmer.

2. Heat oil in large nonstick saucepan over medium heat. Add mushrooms, onion and garlic; cook and stir 5 minutes or until tender.

3. Add rice to mushroom mixture; cook and stir 1 to 2 minutes. Add broth, ½ cup at a time, stirring frequently until broth is absorbed before adding next ½ cup. Continue adding broth and stirring until rice is tender and mixture is creamy, about 20 to 25 minutes.

4. Add chicken, broccoli, tomatoes, parsley, basil, salt and pepper; cook and stir 2 to 3 minutes or until heated through. Sprinkle with cheese.

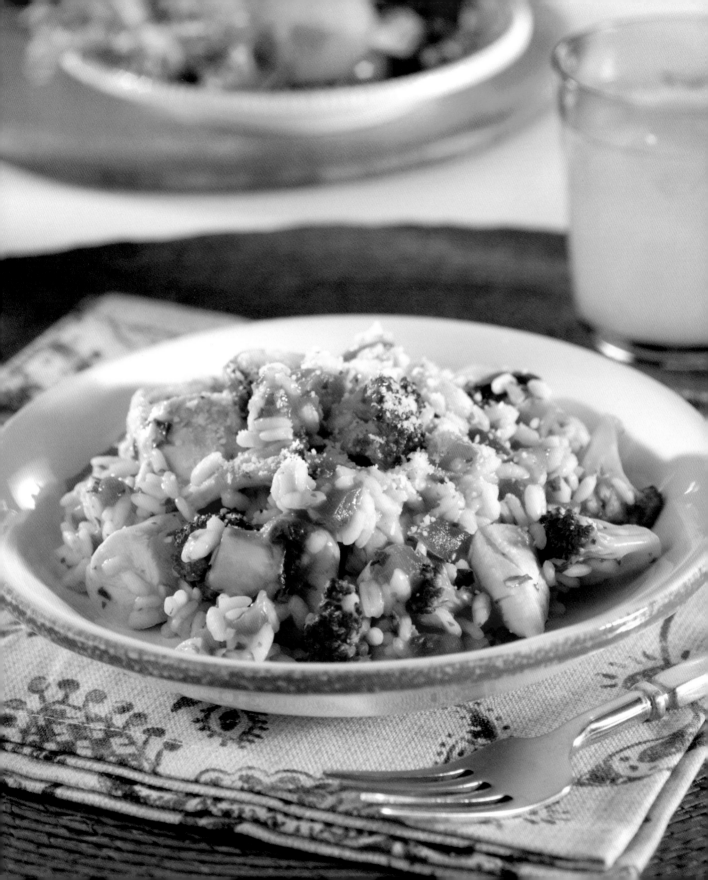

CREAMY LAYERED VEGETABLE BAKE

Makes 8 servings

    2 large eggplants
    4 teaspoons salt, divided
    5 tablespoons olive oil, divided
    2 teaspoons salt, divided
    ½ teaspoon black pepper
    ½ cup chopped onion
    2 medium zucchini, thinly sliced
    1 package (8 ounces) sliced mushrooms
    1 tablespoon Italian seasoning
    2 teaspoons minced garlic, divided
   12 ounces fresh mozzarella cheese, thinly sliced
    1 container (15 ounces) part-skim ricotta cheese
    ¾ cup shredded Parmesan cheese, divided
    1 egg, lightly beaten
    ⅓ cup butter
    3 tablespoons cornstarch
   1¾ cups low-fat (1%) milk

1. Peel eggplants; cut off ends and discard. Cut each eggplant vertically into six equal slices. Place slices in large colander set over bowl; sprinkle with 2 teaspoons salt. Let stand 30 minutes. Rinse eggplant under cold running water. Pat dry with paper towels.

2. Preheat oven to 400°F. Arrange eggplant slices in single layer on baking sheets. Brush both sides of slices evenly with 4 tablespoons oil. Sprinkle evenly with 1 teaspoon salt and pepper. Bake 20 minutes or until golden brown and tender, turning slices halfway through. *Reduce oven temperature to 350°F.* Spray 13×9-inch baking dish with nonstick cooking spray.

3. Meanwhile, heat remaining 1 tablespoon oil in large skillet over medium heat. Add onion; cook and stir 3 minutes. Add zucchini, mushrooms, Italian seasoning, 1 teaspoon garlic and ½ teaspoon salt; cook and stir 5 to 7 minutes or until vegetables are tender.

4. Combine ricotta cheese, ¼ cup Parmesan cheese and egg in medium bowl; mix well.

5. Arrange eggplant slices in single layer in bottom of prepared dish. Layer with half of mozzarella cheese, half of zucchini mixture and half of ricotta mixture. Repeat layers.

continued on page 156

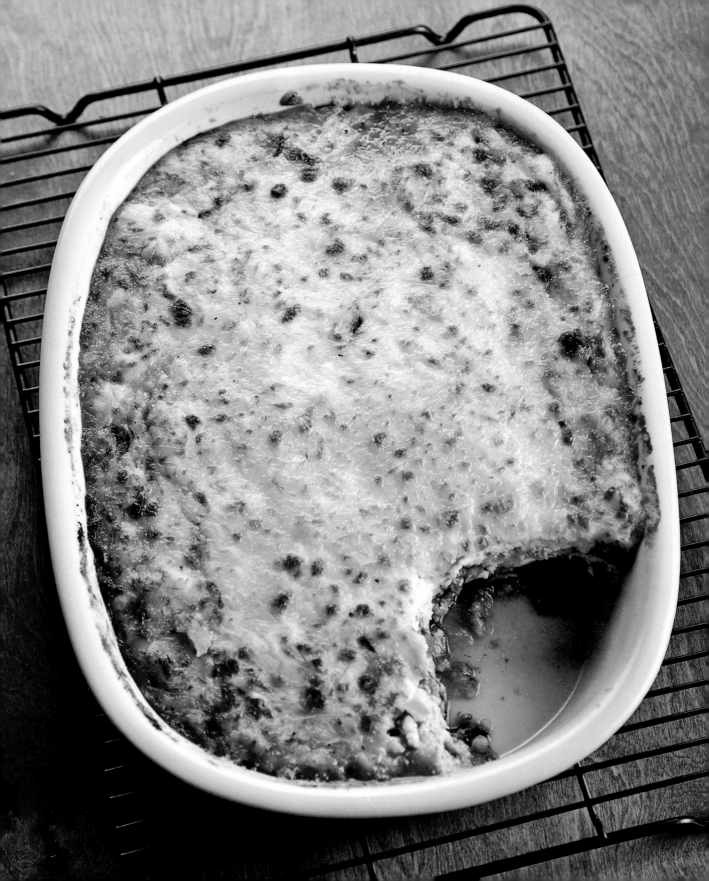

Creamy Layered Vegetable Bake, continued

6. Melt butter in medium saucepan over medium heat. Add remaining 1 teaspoon garlic; cook and stir 1 minute. Whisk in cornstarch; cook 1 minute. Gradually whisk in milk; whisk 2 to 3 minutes or until sauce is thickened. Season with remaining ½ teaspoon salt. Pour sauce evenly over vegetables and cheese. Top with remaining ½ cup Parmesan cheese.

7. Bake 30 minutes or until heated through and cheese is melted. Let stand 10 to 15 minutes before serving.

SALMON WITH BROWN RICE AND VEGETABLES

Makes 4 servings

  2 cups water
12 ounces skinless salmon fillets
  2 cups sliced asparagus (1-inch pieces)
  2 cups cooked brown rice
  1 cup spinach, sliced into ½-inch strips
⅓ cup gluten-free chicken broth
  2 tablespoons chopped fresh chives
  2 tablespoons lemon juice
⅛ teaspoon black pepper

1. Bring water to a boil in large skillet over high heat. Add salmon; reduce heat to medium-low. Cover and simmer 10 minutes or until salmon begins to flake when tested with fork. Remove salmon from skillet; cut into large pieces when cool enough to handle.

2. Spray separate large skillet with nonstick cooking spray; heat over medium-high heat. Add asparagus; cook and stir 6 minutes or until tender. Stir in rice, spinach and broth; reduce heat to low. Cover and cook 1 to 2 minutes or until spinach is wilted and rice is heated through. Stir in salmon, chives, lemon juice and pepper.

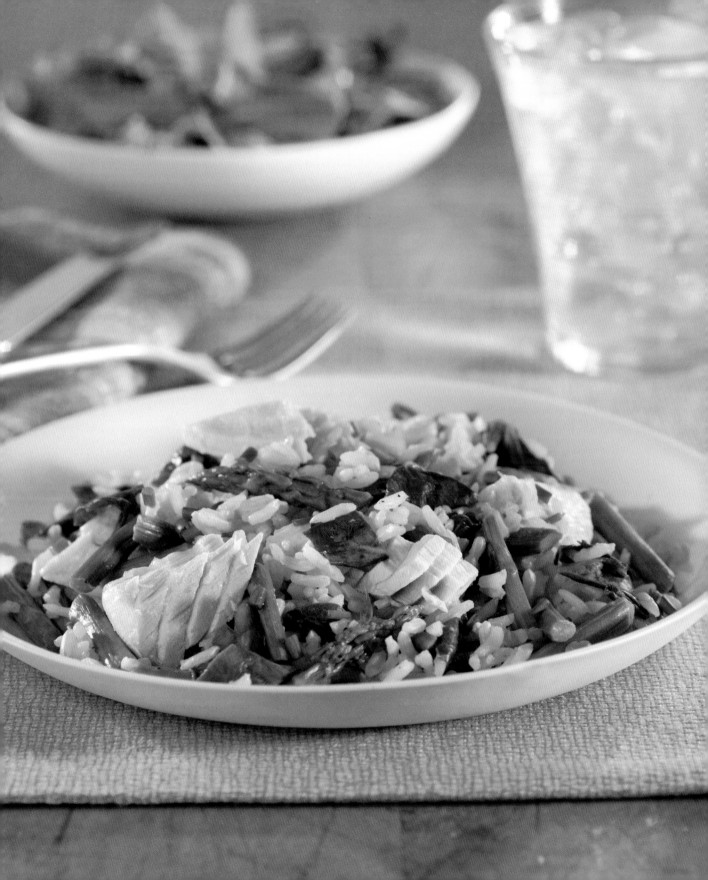

EGGPLANT PARMESAN

Makes 4 servings

    2 egg whites
    2 tablespoons water
    ½ cup crushed gluten-free rice cereal squares
    ¼ cup plus 2 tablespoons grated Parmesan cheese, divided
    1 teaspoon Italian seasoning
    1 large eggplant, peeled and cut into 12 slices (½-inch thick)
    2 teaspoons olive oil
    1 small onion, diced
    1 clove garlic, minced
    2 cans (about 14 ounces each) diced tomatoes
    ½ teaspoon dried basil
    ½ teaspoon dried oregano
    ½ cup (2 ounces) shredded mozzarella cheese

1. Preheat oven to 350°F. Spray 15×10-inch jelly-roll pan with nonstick cooking spray.

2. Whisk egg whites and water in shallow dish. Combine crushed cereal, 2 tablespoons Parmesan cheese and Italian seasoning in another shallow dish. Dip eggplant slices in egg white mixture, letting excess drip back into dish. Coat in cereal mixture, pressing lightly to adhere. Place in single layer in prepared pan.

3. Bake 25 to 30 minutes or until bottoms are browned. Turn slices over; bake 15 to 20 minutes or until well browned and tender.

4. Meanwhile, heat oil in medium nonstick skillet over medium-high heat. Add onion; cook and stir 5 minutes or until softened. Add garlic; cook and stir 1 minute. Stir in tomatoes, basil and oregano; bring to a boil. Reduce heat to low; simmer 15 to 20 minutes or until sauce is thickened, stirring occasionally.

5. Spray 13×9-inch baking dish with nonstick cooking spray. Spread sauce in prepared dish. Arrange eggplant slices in single layer on top of sauce. Sprinkle with mozzarella cheese and remaining ¼ cup Parmesan cheese. Bake 15 to 20 minutes or until sauce is bubbly and cheese is melted.

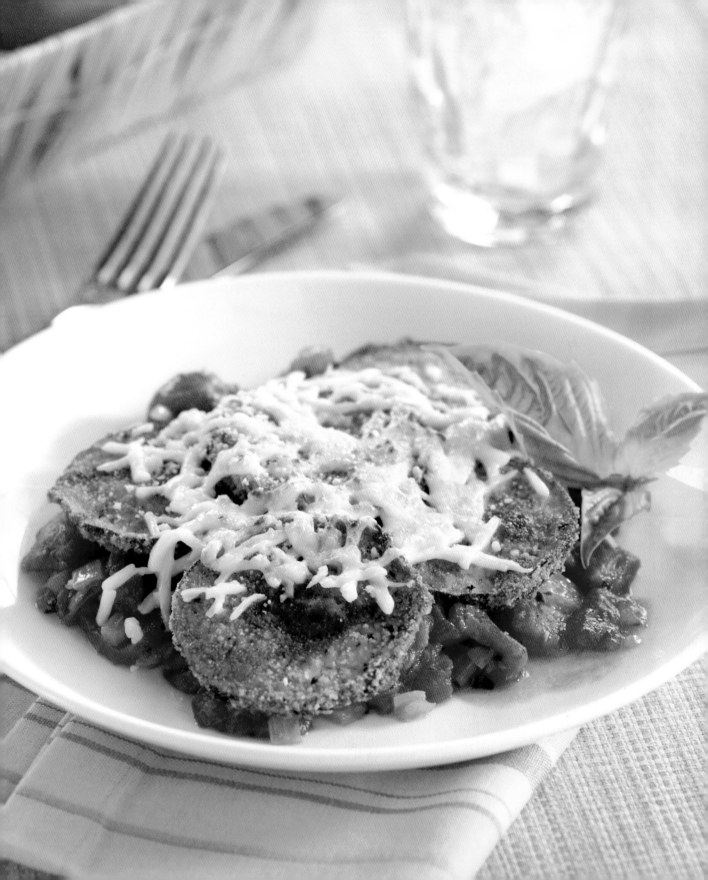

POLENTA LASAGNA

Makes 6 servings

4¼ cups water, divided
1½ cups yellow cornmeal
4 teaspoons finely chopped fresh marjoram
2 medium red bell peppers, chopped
1 teaspoon olive oil
1 pound fresh mushrooms, sliced
1 cup chopped leeks
1 clove garlic, minced
½ cup (2 ounces) shredded part-skim mozzarella cheese
2 tablespoons chopped fresh basil
1 tablespoon chopped fresh oregano
⅛ teaspoon black pepper
¼ cup grated Parmesan cheese, divided

1. Bring 4 cups water to a boil in medium saucepan over high heat. Slowly add cornmeal, stirring constantly. Reduce heat to low; stir in marjoram. Simmer 15 to 20 minutes or until polenta thickens and pulls away from side of pan. Spread in ungreased 13×9-inch baking pan. Cover and chill about 1 hour or until firm.

2. Preheat oven to 350°F. Spray 11×7-inch baking dish with nonstick cooking spray. Place bell peppers and remaining ¼ cup water in food processor or blender; process until smooth.

3. Heat oil in medium nonstick skillet over medium heat. Add mushrooms, leeks and garlic; cook and stir 5 minutes or until leeks are crisp-tender. Stir in mozzarella cheese, basil, oregano and black pepper.

4. Cut cold polenta into 12 (3½-inch) squares; arrange six squares in bottom of prepared dish. Spread with half of bell pepper mixture, half of vegetable mixture and 2 tablespoons Parmesan cheese. Top with remaining six squares of polenta, remaining bell pepper and vegetable mixtures and Parmesan cheese. Bake 20 minutes or until cheese is melted and polenta is golden brown.

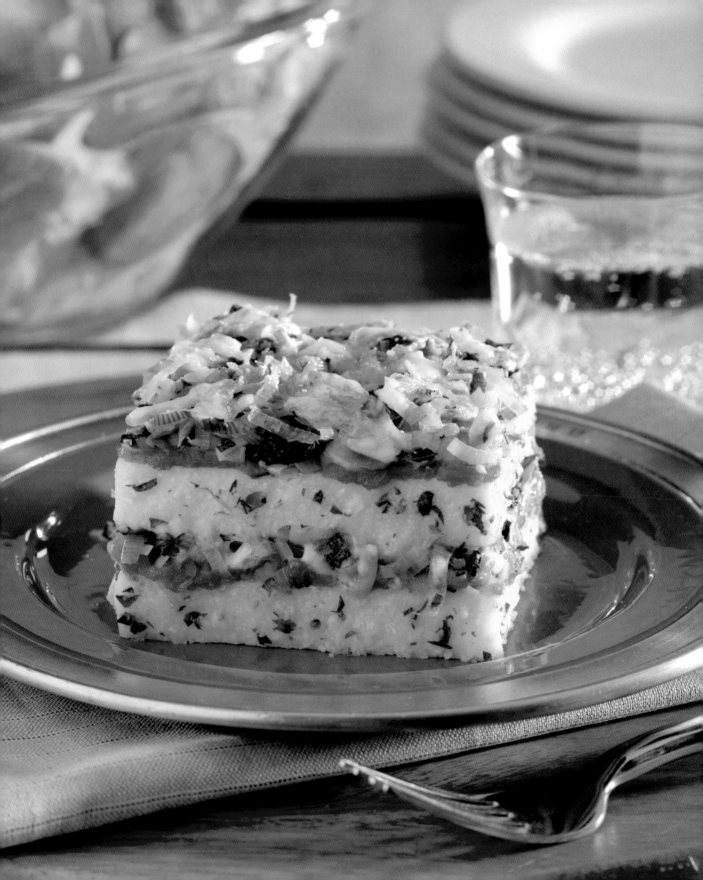

On the Side

TOASTED COCONUT-PECAN SWEET POTATO CASSEROLE

Makes 4 servings

> 2 cans (15 ounces each) sweet potatoes in heavy syrup, drained
> ½ cup (1 stick) butter, softened
> ¼ cup packed brown sugar
> 1 egg
> ½ teaspoon vanilla
> ⅛ teaspoon salt
> ½ cup chopped pecans
> ¼ cup flaked coconut
> 2 tablespoons golden raisins

1. Preheat oven to 325°F. Spray 8-inch square baking dish with nonstick cooking spray.

2. Combine sweet potatoes, butter, brown sugar, egg, vanilla and salt in food processor or blender; process until smooth. Spoon into prepared dish. Sprinkle evenly with pecans, coconut and raisins.

3. Bake 22 to 25 minutes or until heated through and coconut is light golden brown.

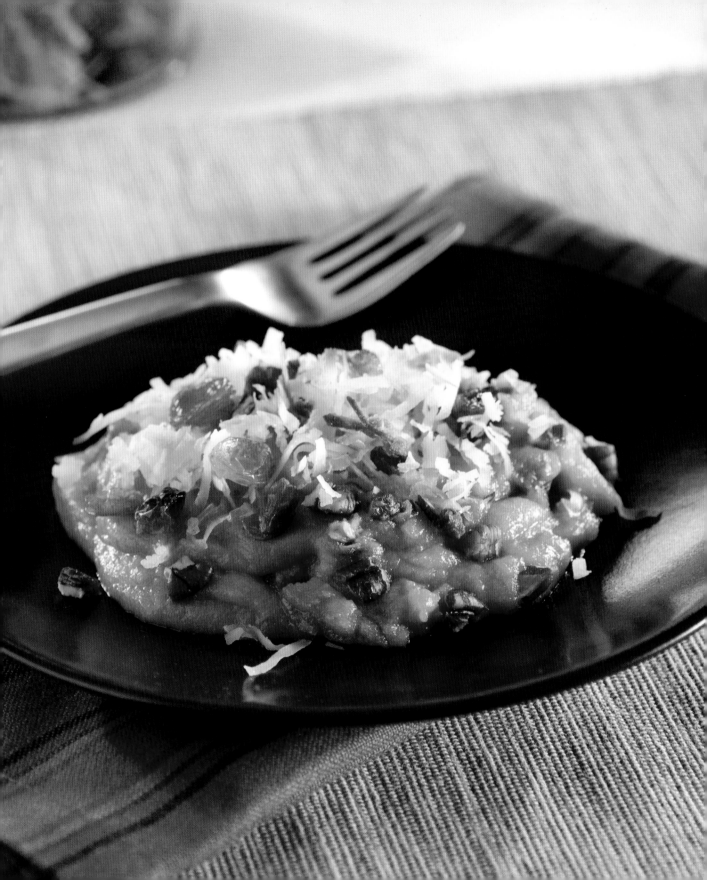

GREEN BEAN CASSEROLE WITH HOMEMADE FRENCH FRIED ONIONS

Makes 6 to 8 servings

> 6 cups water
> 1 pound fresh green beans, cut into 2-inch pieces
> 1 tablespoon vegetable oil
> 8 ounces cremini mushrooms, chopped
> 3 tablespoons butter
> 3 tablespoons rice flour
> 1 teaspoon salt
> ¼ teaspoon red pepper flakes
> 1 cup gluten-free mushroom or vegetable broth
> 1 cup whole milk
> Homemade French Fried Onions (recipe follows)

1. Preheat oven to 350°F. Spray 13×9-inch baking dish with nonstick cooking spray.

2. Bring water to a boil in medium saucepan. Add green beans; cook 4 minutes. Drain.

3. Heat oil in large saucepan over medium heat. Add mushrooms; cook and stir 8 minutes. Add butter; cook and stir until melted. Stir in rice flour, salt and red pepper flakes. Gradually stir in broth and milk; cook and stir until thickened. Remove from heat; stir in green beans. Pour into prepared dish.

4. Bake 30 minutes. Meanwhile, prepare Homemade French Fried Onions.

5. Remove casserole from oven. Top with Homemade French Fried Onions; bake 5 minutes.

HOMEMADE FRENCH FRIED ONIONS

Makes about 1½ cups

> 2 small onions, sliced into rings
> ½ cup whole milk
> ½ cup rice flour
> ½ cup cornmeal
> 1 teaspoon salt
> ½ teaspoon black pepper
> Vegetable oil

continued on page 166

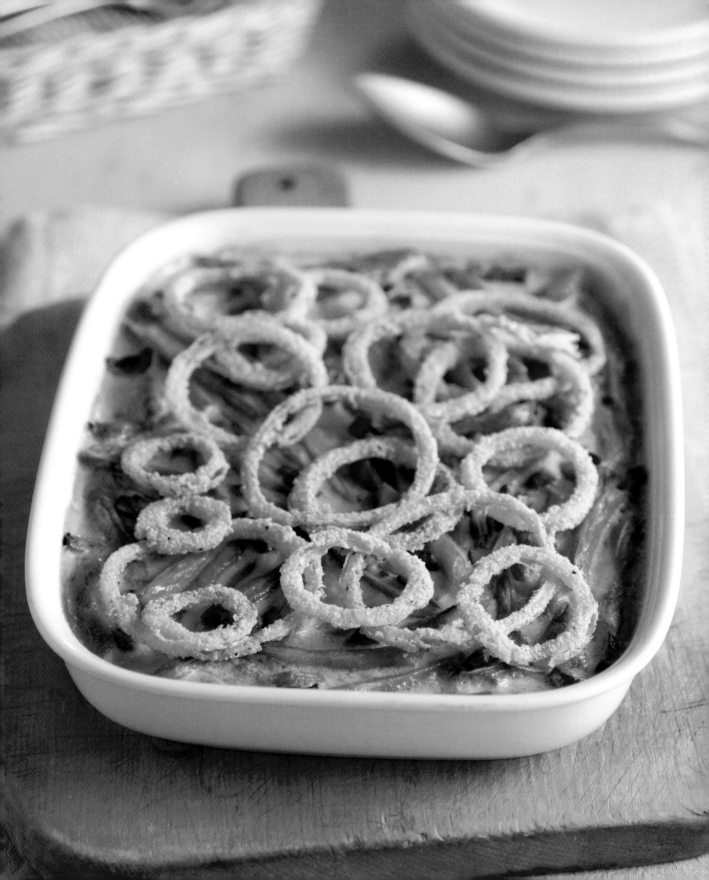

Green Bean Casserole with Homemade French Fried Onions, continued

1. Line baking sheet with paper towels. Separate onion rings and spread in shallow dish. Pour milk over onions; toss to coat. Combine rice flour, cornmeal, salt and pepper in large resealable food storage bag; mix well.

2. Heat oil in large heavy skillet over medium-high heat until temperature registers 300°F to 325°F on deep-fry thermometer.

3. Working in batches, add onion rings to food storage bag; shake to coat. Add onions to oil; fry 2 minutes per side or until golden brown. Remove to prepared baking sheet using slotted spoon. Repeat with remaining onions.

FRUITED CORN PUDDING

Makes 8 servings

    5 cups thawed frozen corn, divided
    5 eggs
    ½ cup milk
  1½ cups whipping cream
    ⅓ cup unsalted butter, melted and cooled
    1 teaspoon vanilla
    ½ teaspoon salt
    ¼ teaspoon ground nutmeg
    3 tablespoons finely chopped dried apricots
    3 tablespoons dried cranberries or raisins
    3 tablespoons finely chopped dates
    2 tablespoons finely chopped dried pear or pineapple

1. Preheat oven to 350°F. Grease 13×9-inch baking dish.

2. Combine 3½ cups corn, eggs and milk in food processor; process until almost smooth.

3. Transfer corn mixture to large bowl. Add cream, butter, vanilla, salt and nutmeg; stir until well blended. Add remaining 1½ cups corn, apricots, cranberries, dates and pears; mix well. Pour into prepared baking dish.

4. Bake 50 to 60 minutes or until center is set and top begins to brown. Let stand 10 to 15 minutes before serving.

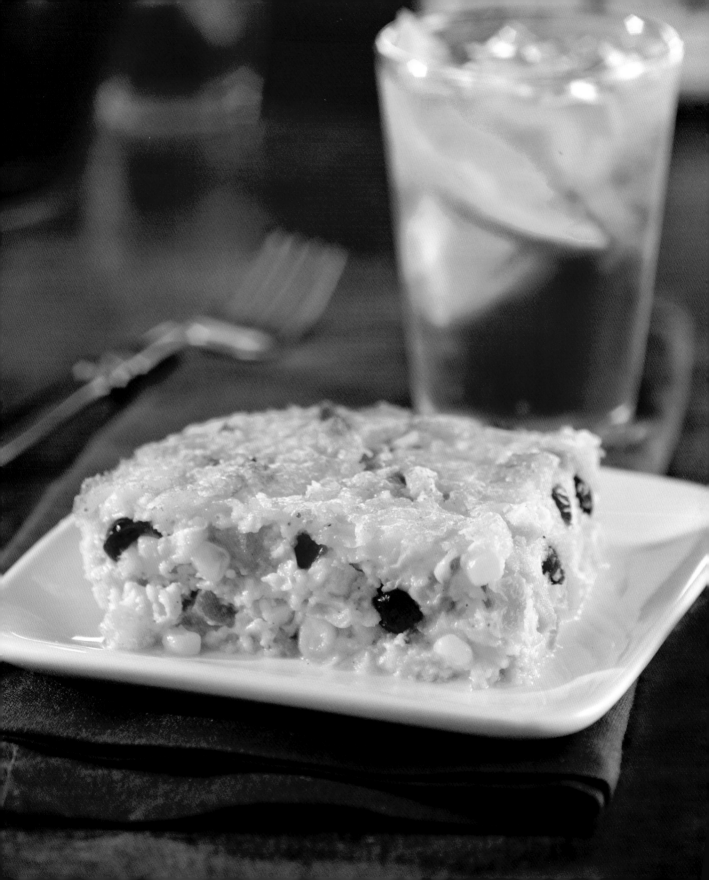

ROASTED CREMINI MUSHROOMS WITH SHALLOTS

Makes 4 servings

>   1 pound cremini mushrooms, halved
>   ½ cup sliced shallots
>   1 tablespoon olive oil
>   ½ teaspoon kosher salt
>   ½ teaspoon dried rosemary
>   ¼ teaspoon black pepper
>   Fresh rosemary (optional)

1. Preheat oven to 400°F.

2. Spread mushrooms and shallots on rimmed baking sheet. Whisk oil, salt, rosemary and pepper in small bowl. Pour over mushrooms and shallots; toss to coat evenly. Arrange in single layer on baking sheet.

3. Bake 15 to 18 minutes or until mushrooms are browned and tender. Garnish with fresh rosemary.

GARLIC AND HERB POLENTA

Makes 6 servings

>   3 tablespoons butter, divided
>   8 cups water
>   2 cups yellow cornmeal
>   2 teaspoons finely minced garlic
>   2 teaspoons salt
>   3 tablespoons chopped fresh herbs such as parsley, chives, thyme or
>   chervil (or a combination)

Slow Cooker Directions

1. Grease inside of slow cooker with 1 tablespoon butter. Add water, cornmeal, remaining 2 tablespoons butter, garlic and salt; mix well. Cover; cook on LOW 4 hours or on HIGH 3 hours, stirring occasionally.

2. Stir in chopped herbs just before serving.

TIP: Polenta may also be poured into a greased pan and allowed to cool until set. Cut into squares or slices, chill until firm and then grill or fry until golden brown.

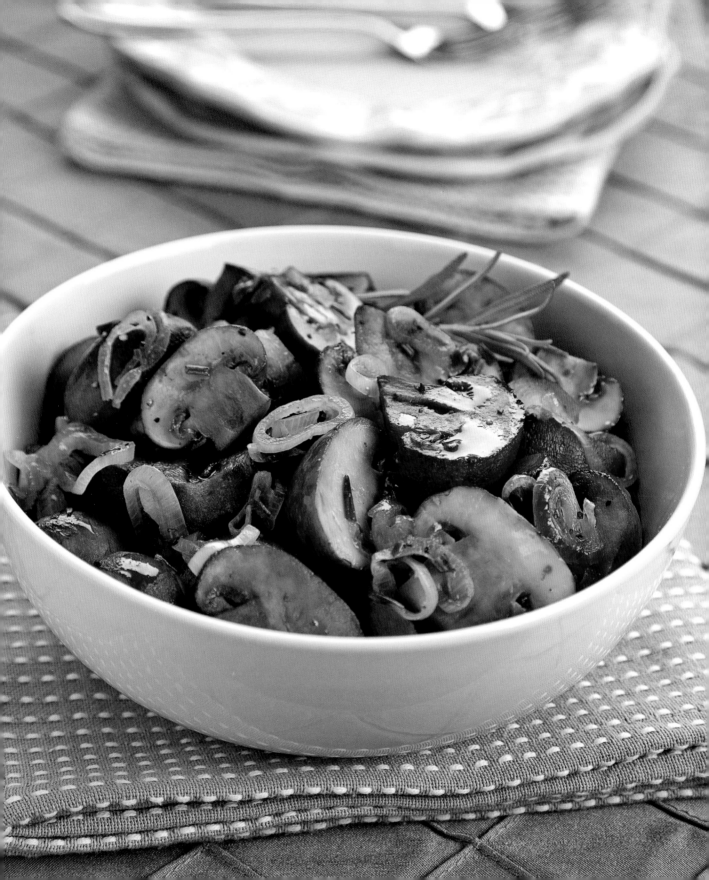

WINTER SQUASH RISOTTO

Makes 4 to 6 servings

2 tablespoons olive oil

1 small butternut squash or medium delicata squash, peeled and cut into
    1-inch pieces (about 2 cups)

1 large shallot or small onion, finely chopped

½ teaspoon paprika

¼ teaspoon dried thyme

¼ teaspoon salt

¼ teaspoon black pepper

1 cup uncooked arborio rice

¼ cup dry white wine

4 to 5 cups gluten-free vegetable broth, warmed

½ cup grated Parmesan or Romano cheese

1. Heat oil in large nonstick skillet over medium heat. Add squash; cook and stir 3 minutes. Add shallot; cook and stir 3 to 4 minutes or until squash is almost tender. Stir in paprika, thyme, salt and pepper. Add rice; stir to coat.

2. Add wine; cook and stir until wine is absorbed. Add broth, ½ cup at a time, stirring frequently until broth is absorbed before adding next ½ cup. Continue adding broth and stirring until rice is tender and mixture is creamy, about 20 to 25 minutes.

3. Sprinkle with cheese just before serving.

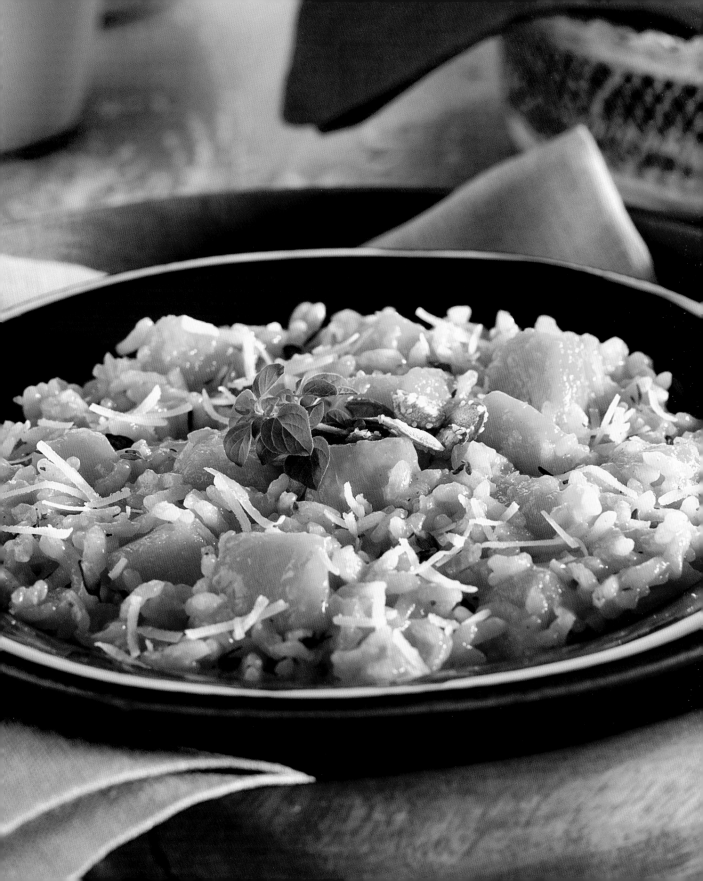

CRISPY OVEN FRIES WITH HERBED DIPPING SAUCE

Makes 3 servings

Herbed Dipping Sauce (recipe follows)
2 large baking potatoes
2 tablespoons vegetable oil
1 teaspoon kosher salt

1. Preheat oven to 425°F. Line two baking sheets with foil; spray with nonstick cooking spray. Prepare Herbed Dipping Sauce; set aside.

2. Cut potatoes lengthwise into ¼-inch slices, then cut each slice into ¼-inch strips. Combine potato strips and oil on prepared baking sheets. Toss to coat evenly; arrange in single layer.

3. Bake 25 minutes. Turn fries over; bake 15 minutes or until light golden brown and crisp. Sprinkle with salt. Serve immediately with Herbed Dipping Sauce.

Herbed Dipping Sauce: Stir ½ cup mayonnaise, 2 tablespoons chopped fresh herbs (such as basil, parsley, oregano and/or dill), 1 teaspoon salt and ½ teaspoon black pepper in small bowl until smooth and well blended. Cover and refrigerate until ready to serve.

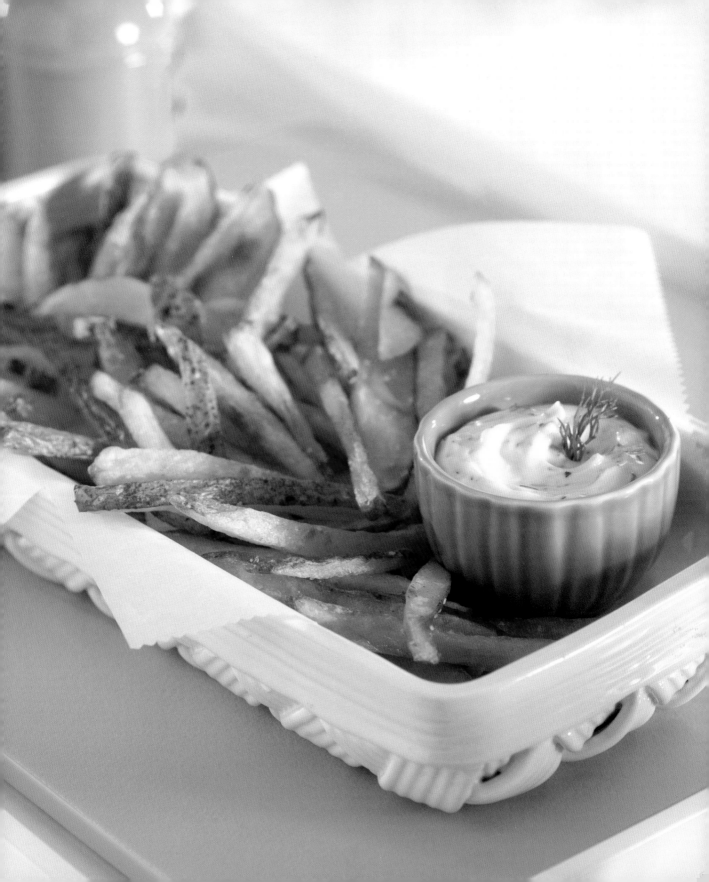

HERBED VEGETABLE KASHA

Makes 8 servings

    1 egg
    1 cup kasha*
    1 tablespoon olive oil
    1 cup chopped broccoli
    1 cup chopped red bell pepper
    ½ cup sliced cremini mushrooms
    ½ cup chopped onion
    2 cloves garlic, minced
    ½ teaspoon dried dill
    ½ teaspoon dried rosemary
    ½ teaspoon dried thyme
    ½ teaspoon salt
    ¼ teaspoon black pepper
    1 cup gluten-free mushroom or vegetable broth

Kasha, or buckwheat groats, is buckwheat that has been toasted. It is commonly found in the Kosher section of the supermarket.

1. Beat egg in medium bowl; add kasha and mix until coated evenly.

2. Heat large nonstick skillet over medium heat; add kasha. Cook and stir 2 to 3 minutes or until kasha is dry and grains are separated. Remove to large bowl; set aside.

3. Heat oil in same skillet over medium heat. Add broccoli, bell pepper, mushrooms, onion and garlic; cook and stir 5 to 7 minutes or until vegetables are crisp-tender. Add dill, rosemary, thyme, salt and pepper; cook and stir 1 minute.

4. Add broth to skillet; bring to a boil. Stir in kasha. Reduce heat to medium-low; cover and cook 10 to 12 minutes or until liquid is absorbed and kasha is tender. Remove from heat. Let stand, covered, 5 minutes. Fluff with fork.

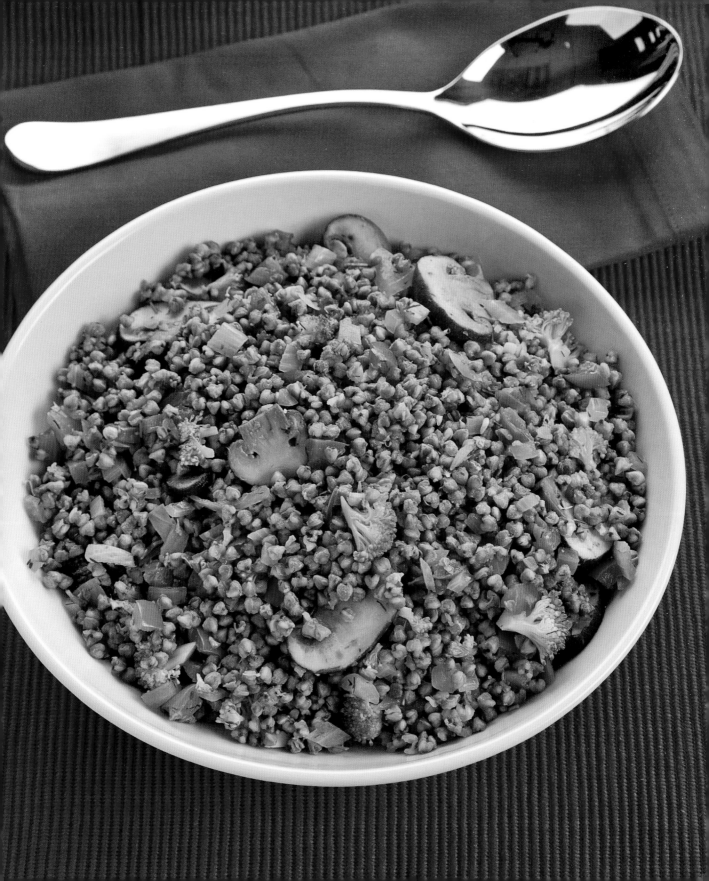

CORN BREAD STUFFING

Makes 12 servings

1½ cups yellow cornmeal
½ cup Gluten-Free All-Purpose Flour Blend (page 19)*
2 tablespoons sugar
2 teaspoons baking powder
1½ teaspoons xanthan gum
½ teaspoon baking soda
½ teaspoon salt
1½ cups low-fat buttermilk
2 egg whites
1 egg
¼ cup (½ stick) butter, melted
3 tablespoons canola or vegetable oil
1 large onion, chopped
½ cup sliced celery
¼ cup chopped fresh sage
¼ cup chopped fresh parsley
¾ cup gluten-free vegetable, chicken or turkey broth

*Or use any all-purpose gluten-free flour blend that does not contain xanthan gum.

1. Preheat oven to 425°F. Spray 8- or 9-inch square baking pan with nonstick cooking spray.

2. For corn bread, combine cornmeal, flour blend, sugar, baking powder, xanthan gum, baking soda and salt in large bowl. Stir in buttermilk, egg whites, egg and butter until well blended. Pour into prepared pan.

3. Bake 25 to 30 minutes or until golden brown and toothpick inserted into center comes out clean. Cool completely in pan on wire rack.**

4. For stuffing, preheat oven to 325°F. Heat oil in large saucepan over medium heat. Add onion and celery; cook 8 to 10 minutes or until vegetables are tender, stirring occasionally. Remove from heat; stir in sage and parsley. Crumble corn bread or cut into cubes. Add to saucepan; gently toss. Slowly stir in broth. Transfer to 13×9-inch baking dish.

5. For moist stuffing, bake, covered, 30 minutes (bake uncovered for drier stuffing).

**Corn bread may be enjoyed on its own or prepared up to 2 days in advance. Store covered at room temperature until ready to use for stuffing.

Variation: For extra flavor or for a festive meal, follow the recipe directions for the stuffing and spoon inside a turkey and roast according to recipe directions.

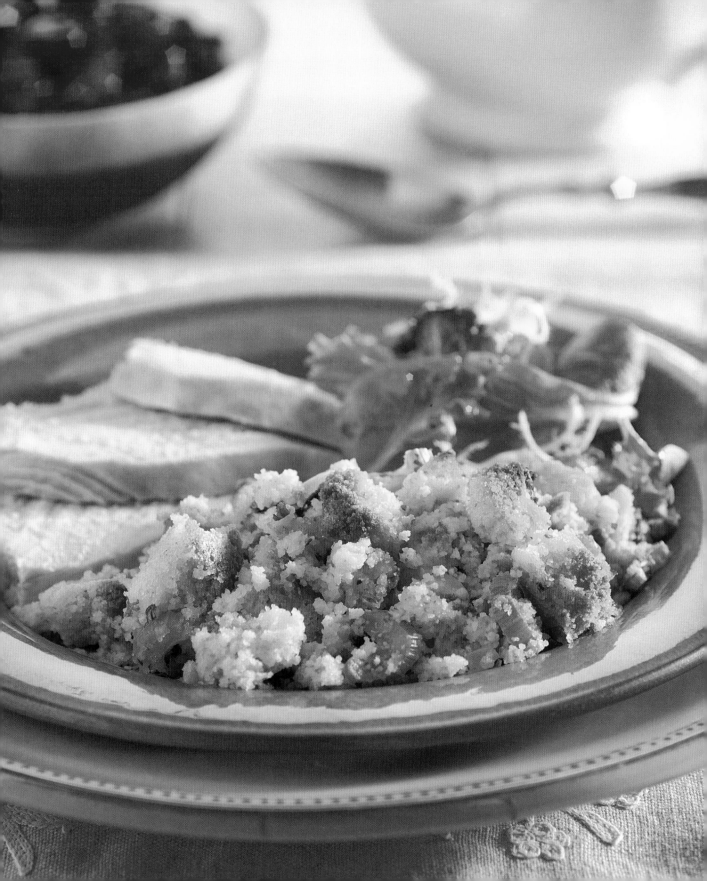

BLACK BEANS WITH BACON AND POBLANO PEPPERS

Makes 4 servings

2 slices bacon
2 medium poblano peppers, chopped (about 1 cup)
1 small onion, chopped
2 cloves garlic, minced
1 teaspoon salt, divided
½ teaspoon chili powder
1 can (about 15 ounces) black beans, rinsed and drained
⅓ cup water

1. Cook bacon in large skillet over medium-high heat 6 to 7 minutes or until crisp, turning occasionally. Transfer to paper towel-lined plate. Chop bacon; set aside.

2. Combine poblano, onion, garlic, ½ teaspoon salt and chili powder in same skillet. Cook and stir 5 minutes or until crisp-tender. Add black beans, water and remaining ½ teaspoon salt; cook 10 minutes or until liquid is absorbed and vegetables are tender.

3. Stir bacon into bean mixture just before serving.

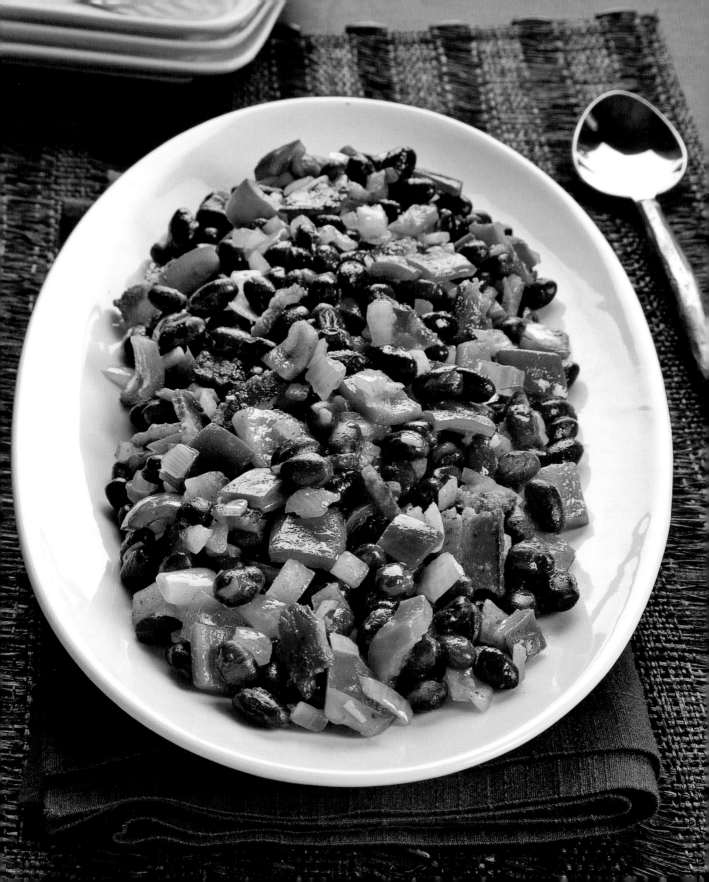

POTATO-ZUCCHINI PANCAKES

Makes 6 pancakes (about 3 servings)

  1 medium unpeeled baking potato, shredded
  ½ small zucchini, shredded
  1 green onion, thinly sliced, plus additional for garnish
  1 egg, lightly beaten
  2 tablespoons rice flour
    Vegetable oil
    Sour cream (optional)

1. Combine potato, zucchini, 1 green onion, egg and rice flour in medium bowl; mix well.

2. Heat ¼ inch of oil in large heavy skillet over medium heat. Drop potato mixture into skillet by ⅓ cupfuls. Flatten pancakes with spatula; cook about 5 minutes per side or until browned.

3. Serve with sour cream and top with additional green onion, if desired.

TIP

For a sweeter version, try using sweet potatoes and carrots. Top with applesauce, if desired.

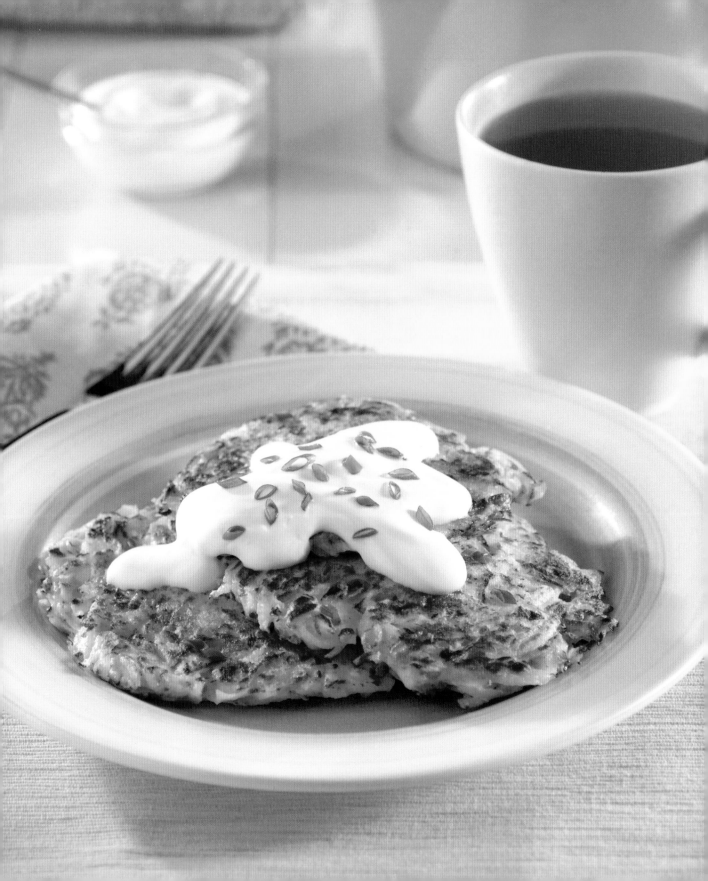

MILLET PILAF

Makes 6 servings

    1 tablespoon olive oil
    ½ onion, finely chopped
    ½ red bell pepper, finely chopped
    1 carrot, finely chopped
    2 cloves garlic, minced
    1 cup uncooked millet
    3 cups water
      Grated peel and juice of 1 lemon
    ¾ teaspoon salt
    ¼ teaspoon black pepper
    2 tablespoons chopped fresh parsley (optional)

1. Heat oil in medium saucepan over medium heat. Add onion, bell pepper, carrot and garlic; cook and stir 5 minutes or until softened. Add millet; cook and stir 5 minutes or until lightly toasted.

2. Stir in water, lemon peel, lemon juice, salt and black pepper; bring to a boil. Reduce heat to low; cover and simmer 30 minutes or until water is absorbed and millet is tender. Cover and let stand 5 minutes. Fluff with fork. Sprinkle with parsley, if desired.

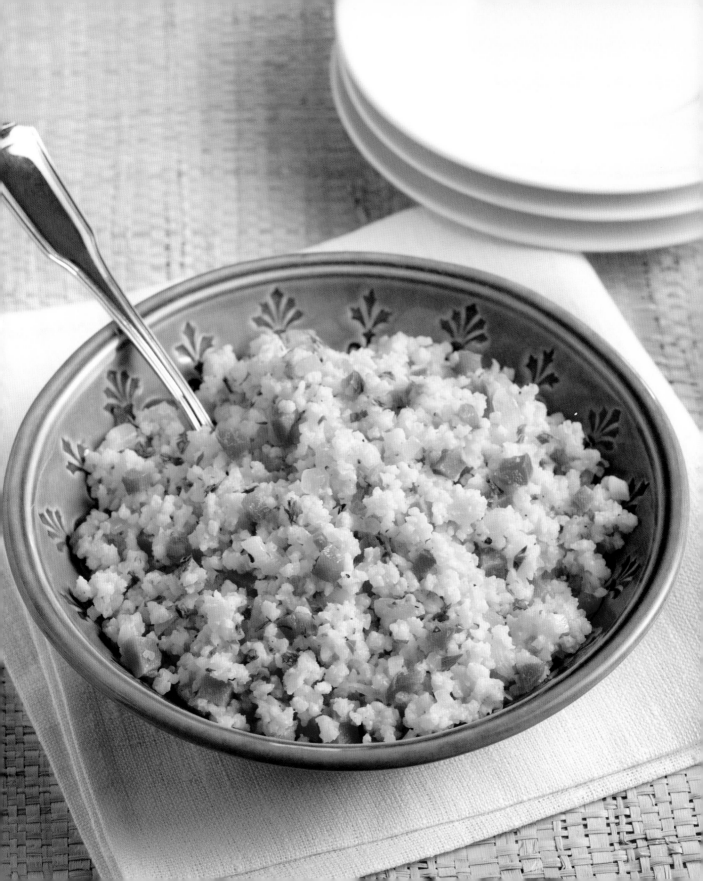

SAVORY CORN CAKES

Makes 12 cakes (4 to 6 servings)

  1 cup Gluten-Free All-Purpose Flour Blend (page 19)*
  1 cup yellow cornmeal
  1 teaspoon baking powder
  1 teaspoon salt
  2 cups frozen corn, thawed
  1 cup (4 ounces) shredded smoked Cheddar cheese
  1 cup low-fat buttermilk
  2 eggs
  3 green onions, finely chopped
  2 cloves garlic, minced
  2 tablespoons chili powder
  2 tablespoons vegetable oil
    Salsa and lime wedges (optional)

*Or use any all-purpose gluten-free flour blend that does not contain xanthan gum.

1. Combine flour blend, cornmeal, baking powder and salt in large bowl; mix well. Stir in corn, cheese, buttermilk, eggs, green onions, garlic and chili powder until well combined.

2. Heat oil in large nonstick skillet over medium-high heat. Drop batter by ¼ cupfuls into skillet. Cook 3 minutes per side or until golden brown. Serve with salsa, if desired. Garnish with lime wedges. Serve immediately.

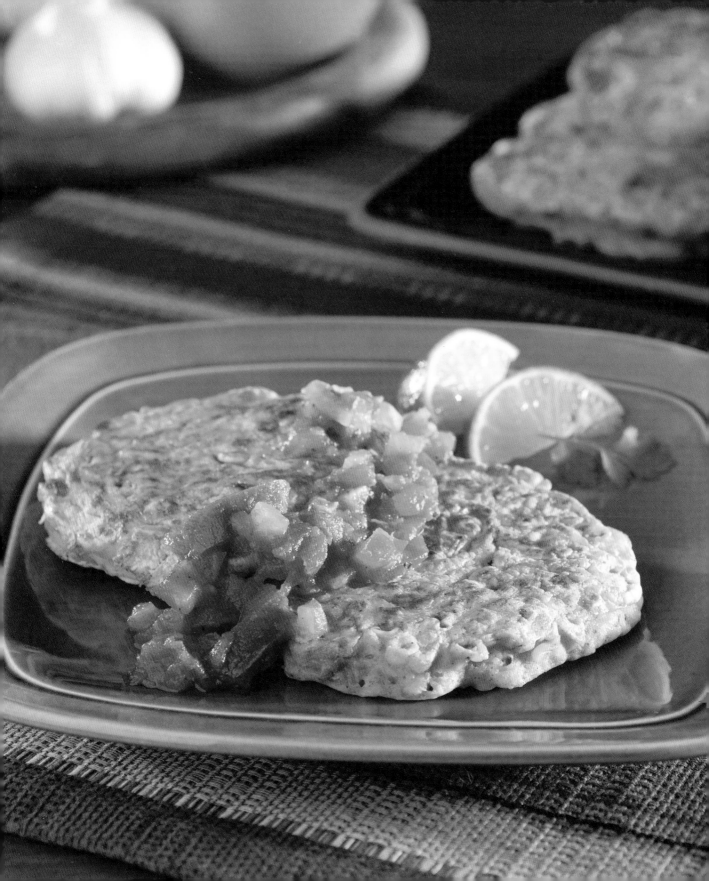

Family Favorites

BEEF & TURKEY MEAT LOAF

¾ pound ground beef
¾ pound ground turkey
½ cup grated carrot
⅓ cup finely chopped onion
⅓ cup crushed gluten-free corn or rice cereal squares
⅓ cup plus 2 tablespoons gluten-free chili sauce, divided
1 egg, beaten
¾ teaspoon salt
½ teaspoon black pepper

1. Preheat oven to 350°F.

2. Combine beef, turkey, carrot, onion, cereal, ⅓ cup chili sauce, egg, salt and pepper in large bowl; mix well.

3. Shape into 8-inch-long loaf in 13×9-inch pan. Spread remaining 2 tablespoons chili sauce evenly over top of meat loaf.

4. Bake 1 hour and 15 minutes or until cooked through (165°F).

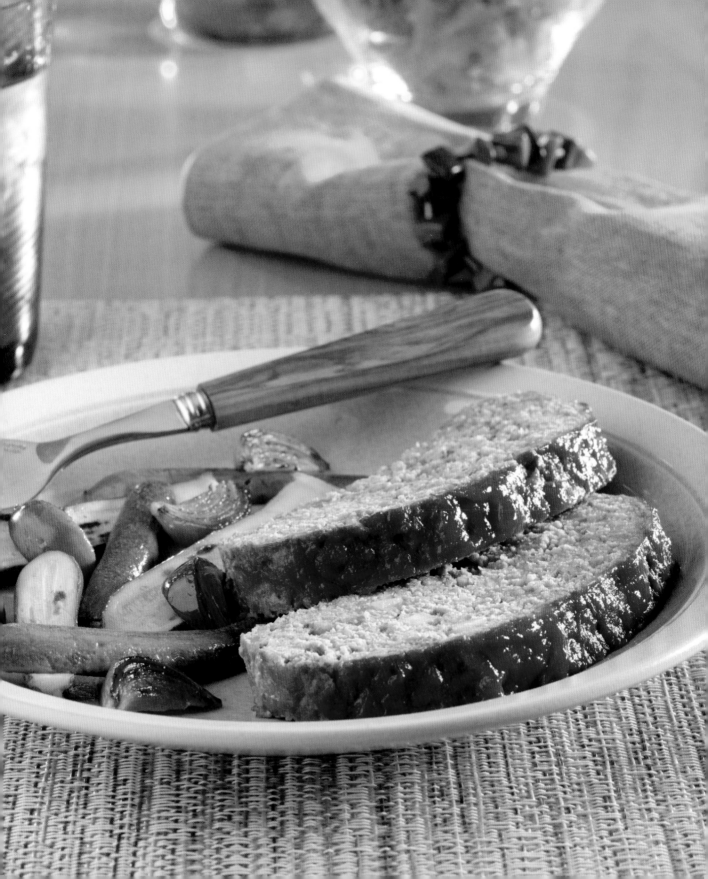

SWEET POTATO SHEPHERD'S PIE

Makes 6 servings

    1 large sweet potato, peeled and cubed
    1 large russet potato, peeled and cubed
    ½ to 1 cup milk
 1½ teaspoons salt, divided
    2 cups gluten-free chicken broth
    3 tablespoons rice flour
    1 teaspoon cider vinegar
    1 teaspoon dried thyme
    ½ teaspoon dried sage
    ½ teaspoon black pepper
    1 pound ground turkey
    2 packages (4 ounces each) sliced mixed mushrooms *or* 8 ounces sliced
            cremini mushrooms
    1 tablespoon minced garlic
    ¾ cup frozen peas, thawed

1. Place potatoes in medium saucepan. Cover with water; bring to a boil over medium-high heat. Reduce heat; cover and simmer 20 minutes or until potatoes are very tender. Drain potatoes; return to saucepan. Mash with potato masher; stir in enough milk until desired consistency is reached and ½ teaspoon salt.

2. Heat broth in small saucepan over medium heat. Whisk in rice flour; cook and stir 2 minutes. Reduce heat to low; cook until thickened. Stir in vinegar, thyme, remaining 1 teaspoon salt, sage and pepper.

3. Spray large nonstick ovenproof skillet with nonstick cooking spray. Add turkey, mushrooms and garlic; cook and stir over medium-high heat until turkey is no longer pink and mushrooms begin to give off liquid.

4. Pour gravy into skillet; simmer 5 minutes. Add peas; cook and stir until heated through. Remove from heat. Spoon potato mixture over turkey mixture; spray with cooking spray.

5. Preheat broiler. Broil 4 to 5 inches from heat source 5 minutes or until mixture is heated through and potatoes begin to brown.

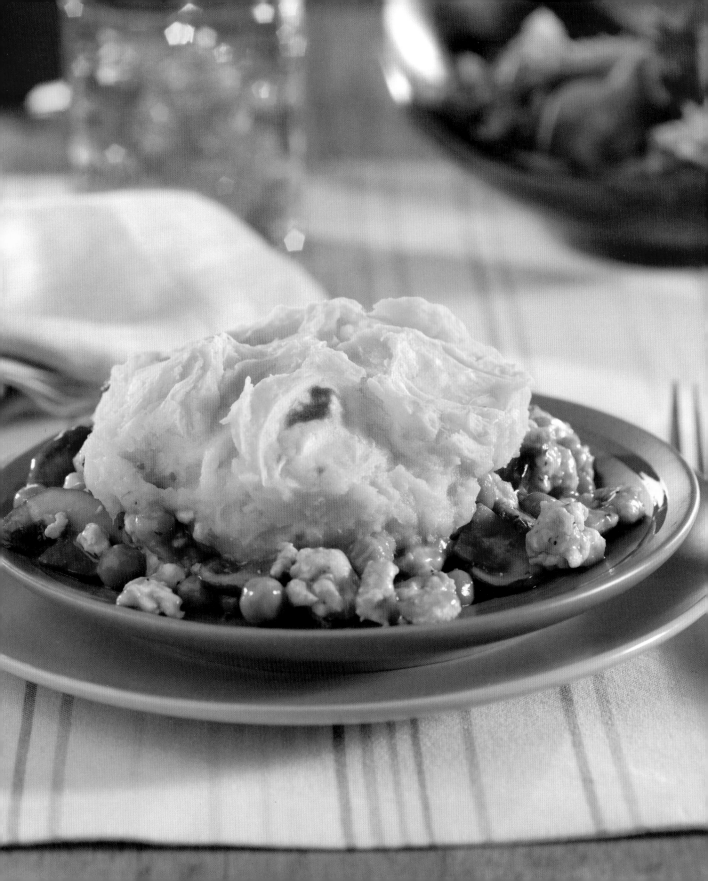

BETTER-THAN-TAKE-OUT FRIED RICE

Makes 4 servings

> 3 tablespoons gluten-free soy sauce
> 1 tablespoon unseasoned rice vinegar
> ⅛ teaspoon red pepper flakes
> 1 red bell pepper
> 1 tablespoon peanut or vegetable oil
> 6 green onions, cut into 1-inch pieces
> 1 tablespoon grated fresh ginger
> 1½ teaspoons minced garlic
> ½ pound boneless pork loin or tenderloin, cut into 1-inch pieces
> 2 cups shredded coleslaw mix
> 1 package (about 8 ounces) cooked whole grain brown rice

1. Whisk soy sauce, vinegar and red pepper flakes in small bowl until well blended.

2. Cut bell pepper into decorative shapes using 1¼- to 1½-inch cookie cutters or cut into 1-inch pieces.

3. Heat oil in large nonstick skillet or wok over medium-high heat. Add bell pepper, green onions, ginger and garlic; stir-fry 1 minute. Add pork; stir-fry 2 to 3 minutes or until pork is barely pink.

4. Stir in coleslaw mix, rice and soy sauce mixture; cook and stir 1 minute or until heated through.

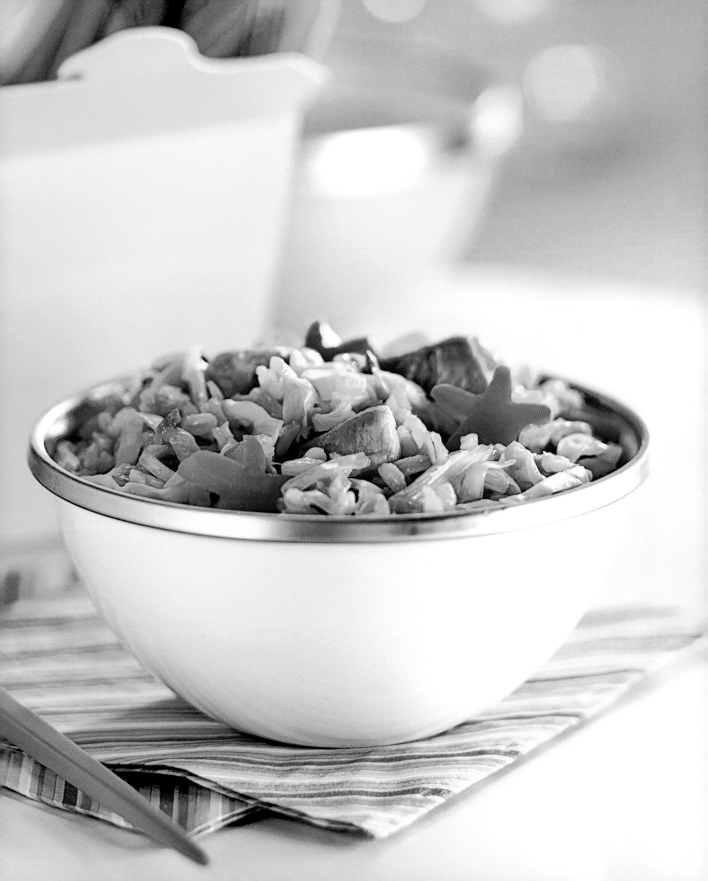

CLASSIC CHILI

Makes 6 servings

    1½ pounds ground beef
    1½ cups chopped onion
      1 cup chopped green bell pepper
      2 cloves garlic, minced
      3 cans (about 15 ounces each) dark red kidney beans, rinsed and drained
      2 cans (about 15 ounces each) tomato sauce
      1 can (about 14 ounces) diced tomatoes
      2 to 3 teaspoons chili powder
      1 to 2 teaspoons dry hot mustard
     ¾ teaspoon dried basil
     ½ teaspoon black pepper
      1 to 2 dried hot chile peppers (optional)
        Shredded Cheddar cheese (optional)
        Fresh cilantro leaves (optional)

Slow Cooker Directions

1. Cook and stir beef, onion, bell pepper and garlic in large skillet over medium-high heat 6 to 8 minutes or until beef is browned and onion is tender. Drain fat. Transfer to slow cooker.

2. Add beans, tomato sauce, diced tomatoes, chili powder, mustard, basil, black pepper and chile peppers, if desired, to slow cooker; mix well. Cover; cook on LOW 8 to 10 hours or on HIGH 4 to 5 hours. Remove and discard chiles before serving. Top with cheese, if desired. Garnish with cilantro.

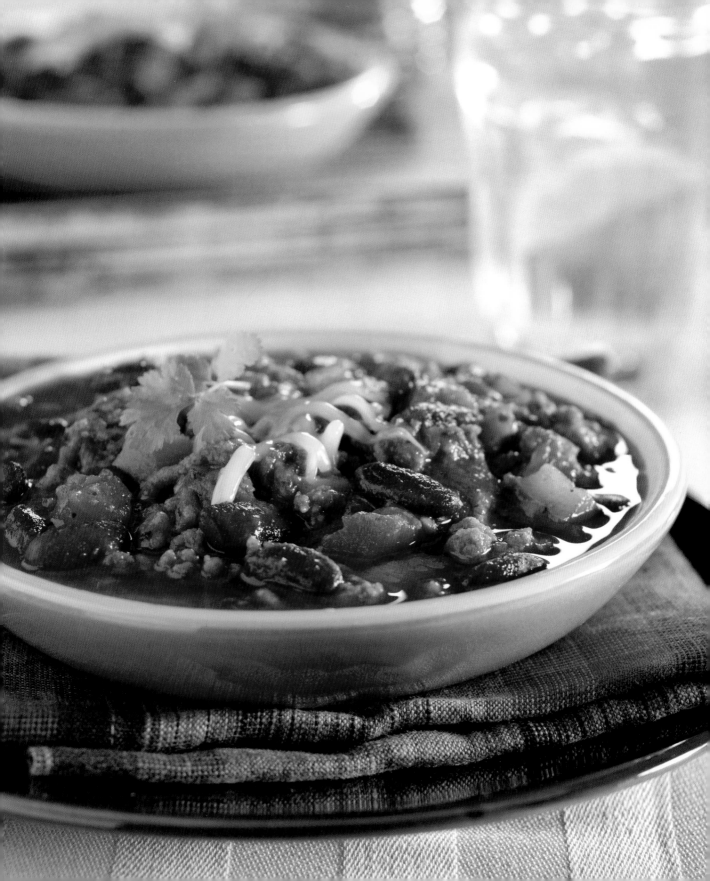

PARMESAN-CRUSTED CHICKEN

Makes 4 servings

    4 boneless skinless chicken breasts (about 4 ounces each)
    ¼ cup grated Parmesan cheese
    ¼ cup Gluten-Free All-Purpose Flour Blend (page 19)*
    2 teaspoons Italian seasoning
    ½ teaspoon salt
    ½ teaspoon black pepper
    2 tablespoons olive oil

*Or use any all-purpose gluten-free flour blend that does not contain xanthan gum.

1. Pound chicken breasts between sheets of waxed paper using meat mallet to ¼-inch thickness. Combine cheese, flour blend, Italian seasoning, salt and pepper in large resealable food storage bag.

2. Add one chicken breast to bag at a time; shake to coat evenly. Heat oil in large nonstick skillet over medium heat. Cook chicken in single layer 4 to 5 minutes per side or until golden brown and no longer pink.

TIP

Serve this savory dish with assorted vegetables like broccoli and carrots.

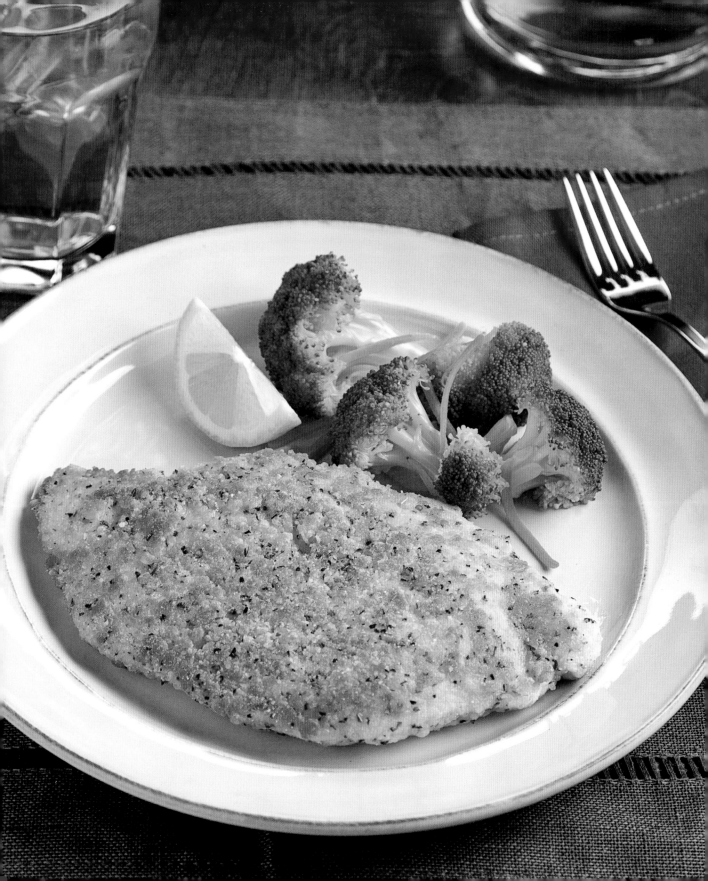

SPEEDY SALMON PATTIES

Makes 6 patties (about 3 servings)

    1 can (12 ounces) pink salmon, undrained
    1 egg, lightly beaten
    ¼ cup minced green onions
    1 tablespoon chopped fresh dill
    1 clove garlic, minced
    ½ cup rice flour
  1½ teaspoons baking powder
    Vegetable oil

1. Drain salmon, reserving 2 tablespoons liquid. Place salmon in medium bowl; break apart with fork. Add reserved liquid, egg, green onions, dill and garlic; mix well.

2. Combine rice flour and baking powder in small bowl. Add to salmon mixture; mix well. Shape into six patties.

3. Heat ¾ inch oil in large heavy skillet or Dutch over medium-high heat to 350°F.

4. Add salmon patties; cook on both sides until golden brown, turning once. Remove using slotted spoon; drain on paper towels. Serve immediately.

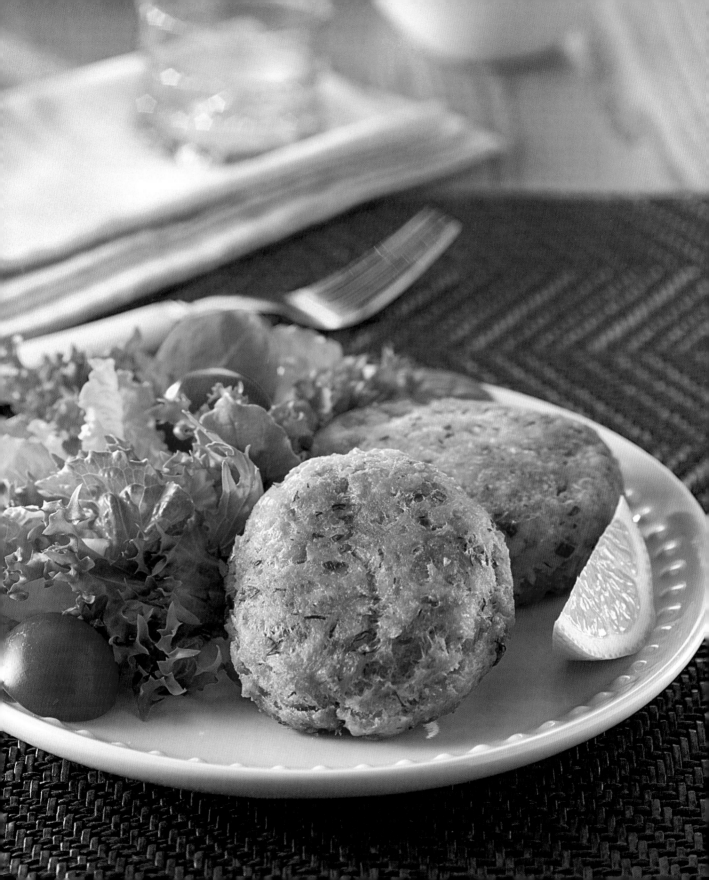

VEGETABLE ENCHILADAS

Makes 6 servings

   1 tablespoon vegetable oil
   2 large poblano peppers or green bell peppers, cut into 2-inch strips
   1 large zucchini, cut into 2-inch strips
   1 large red onion, sliced
   1 cup sliced mushrooms
   1 teaspoon ground cumin
   1 pound fresh tomatillos (about 8 large), peeled
  ½ to 1 jalapeño pepper*
   1 clove garlic
  ½ teaspoon salt
   1 cup loosely packed fresh cilantro, plus additional for garnish
  12 corn tortillas, warmed to soften
   2 cups (8 ounces) shredded Mexican cheese blend, divided

*Jalapeño peppers can sting and irritate the skin, so wear rubber gloves when handling peppers and do not touch your eyes.

1. Preheat oven to 400°F.

2. Heat oil in large nonstick skillet over medium heat. Add poblano peppers, zucchini, onion, mushrooms and cumin; cook and stir 8 to 10 minutes or until vegetables are crisp-tender.

3. Meanwhile, place tomatillos in large microwavable bowl. Cover with vented plastic wrap. Microwave on HIGH 6 to 7 minutes or until very tender.

4. Combine tomatillos with juice, jalapeño, garlic and salt in food processor or blender; process until smooth. Add 1 cup cilantro; pulse until combined and cilantro is coarsely chopped.

5. Divide vegetables evenly among tortillas. Spoon heaping tablespoon of cheese in center of each tortilla; roll up to enclose filling. Place in 13×9-inch baking dish. Pour sauce evenly over enchiladas. Sprinkle with remaining 1 cup cheese.

6. Bake, covered, 18 to 20 minutes or until cheese is melted and enchiladas are heated through. Garnish with additional cilantro. Serve immediately.

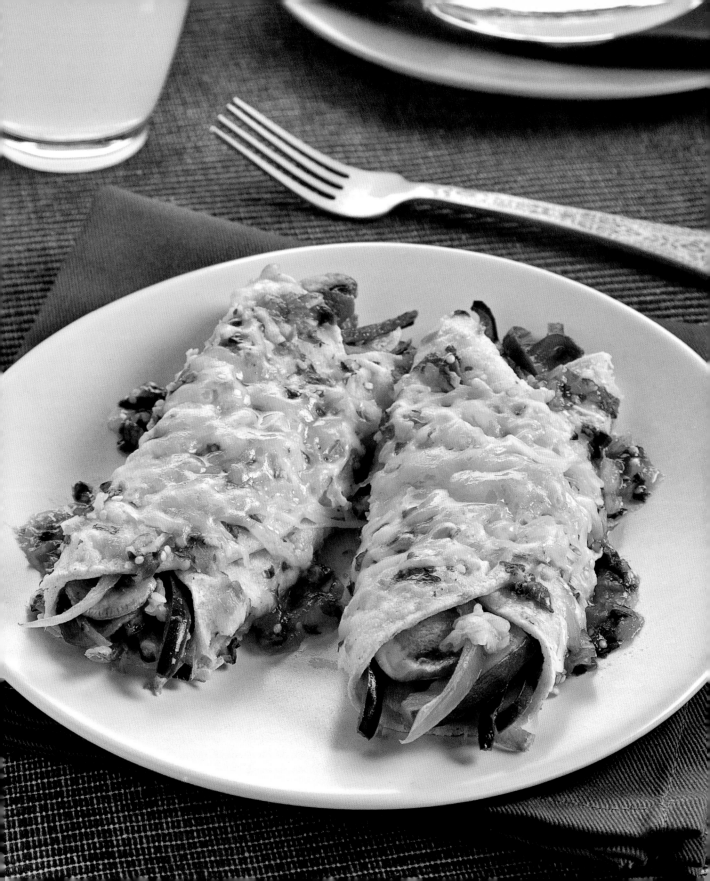

SWEET AND SOUR CHICKEN

Makes 4 servings

2 tablespoons unseasoned rice vinegar
2 tablespoons gluten-free soy sauce
3 cloves garlic, minced
½ teaspoon minced fresh ginger
¼ teaspoon red pepper flakes (optional)
6 ounces boneless skinless chicken breasts, cut into ½-inch strips
1 teaspoon vegetable oil
3 green onions, cut into 1-inch pieces
1 large green bell pepper, cut into 1-inch pieces
1 tablespoon cornstarch
½ cup gluten-free chicken broth
2 tablespoons apricot fruit spread
1 can (11 ounces) mandarin orange segments, drained
2 cups hot cooked white rice

1. Whisk vinegar, soy sauce, garlic, ginger and red pepper flakes, if desired, in medium bowl until smooth and well blended. Add chicken; toss to coat. Marinate 20 minutes at room temperature.

2. Heat oil in wok or large nonstick skillet over medium heat. Drain chicken; reserve marinade. Add chicken to wok; stir-fry 3 minutes. Stir in green onions and bell pepper.

3. Stir cornstarch into reserved marinade until well blended. Stir broth, fruit spread and marinade mixture into wok. Bring to a boil; cook and stir 2 minutes or until chicken is cooked through and sauce is thickened. Add oranges; cook until heated through. Serve over rice.

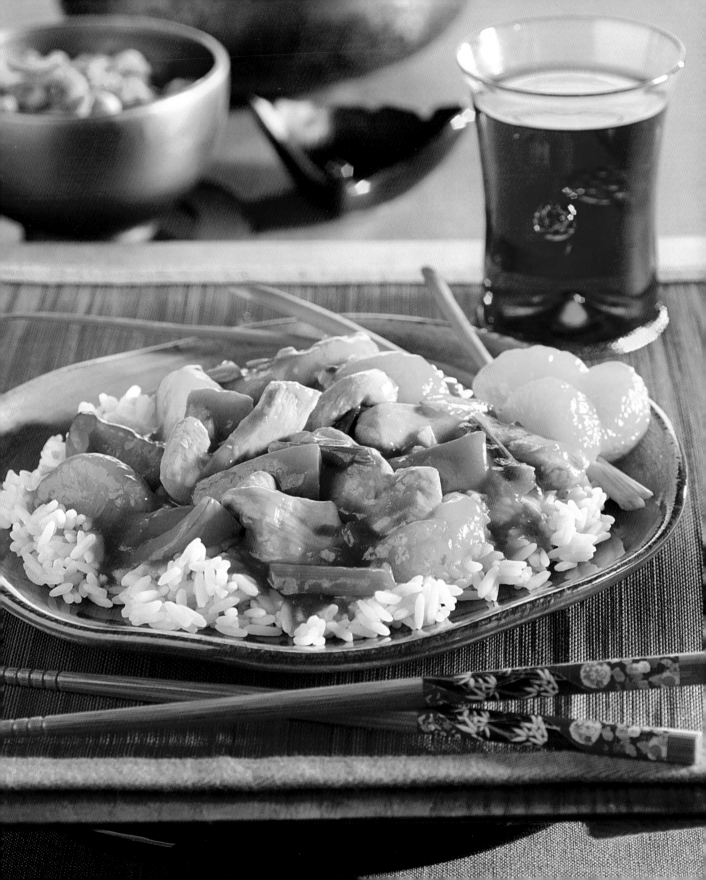

FAMILY-STYLE FRANKFURTERS WITH RICE AND RED BEANS

Makes 6 servings

1 tablespoon vegetable oil
1 onion, chopped
½ green bell pepper, chopped
2 cloves garlic, minced
1 can (about 15 ounces) red kidney beans, rinsed and drained
1 can (about 15 ounces) Great Northern beans, rinsed and drained
½ pound gluten-free beef frankfurters, cut into ¼-inch-thick pieces
1 cup uncooked instant brown rice
1 cup gluten-free vegetable broth
¼ cup packed brown sugar
¼ cup ketchup
3 tablespoons dark molasses
1 tablespoon Dijon mustard

1. Preheat oven to 350°F. Spray 13×9-inch baking dish with nonstick cooking spray.

2. Heat oil in large saucepan or Dutch oven over medium-high heat. Add onion, bell pepper and garlic; cook and stir 2 minutes or until tender.

3. Add beans, frankfurters, rice, broth, brown sugar, ketchup, molasses and mustard to saucepan; gently mix. Transfer to prepared baking dish.

4. Bake, covered, 30 minutes or until rice is tender.

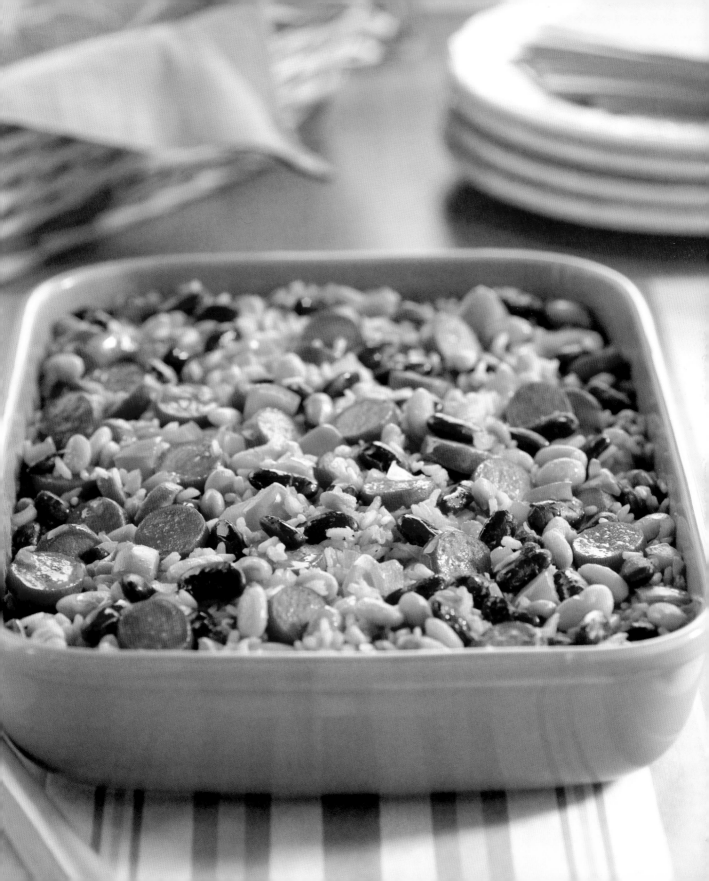

PAN-FRIED GNOCCHI SKILLET

Makes 6 servings

　　1 pound baking potatoes (about 2 medium), cut into 1-inch pieces
　　¼ cup grated Parmesan cheese
　　3 tablespoons rice flour, plus additional for work surface
　　1 egg
　　1 egg white
　　½ teaspoon salt
　　1 tablespoon olive oil
　　¾ pound bulk hot Italian sausage, casings removed
　　2 large zucchini, diced
　　1 cup sliced cremini mushrooms
　　1 can (about 14 ounces) diced tomatoes with basil, garlic and oregano, drained

1. Place potatoes in large microwavable bowl. Cover; microwave on HIGH 8 to 10 minutes or until very tender. Cool 10 minutes. Peel potatoes.

2. Meanwhile, combine cheese, 3 tablespoons rice flour, egg, egg white and salt in medium bowl; mix well. Mash or press potatoes through ricer into cheese mixture in medium bowl.

3. Heavily dust cutting board or work surface with rice flour. Working in batches, scoop portions of dough onto board and roll into ½-inch-thick rope using rice-floured hands. Cut each rope into ¾-inch pieces. Cover unrolled dough with damp paper towel to keep from drying out.

4. Heat oil in large nonstick skillet over medium heat. Working in batches, add gnocchi in single layer and cook 5 minutes per side until lightly browned and heated through, turning once. Keep warm.

5. Cook sausage in same skillet over medium-high heat 8 to 10 minutes or until no longer pink, stirring to break up meat. Add zucchini and mushrooms; cook and stir 3 to 5 minutes or until crisp-tender. Add tomatoes; cook until heated through. Add gnocchi to skillet; gently toss.

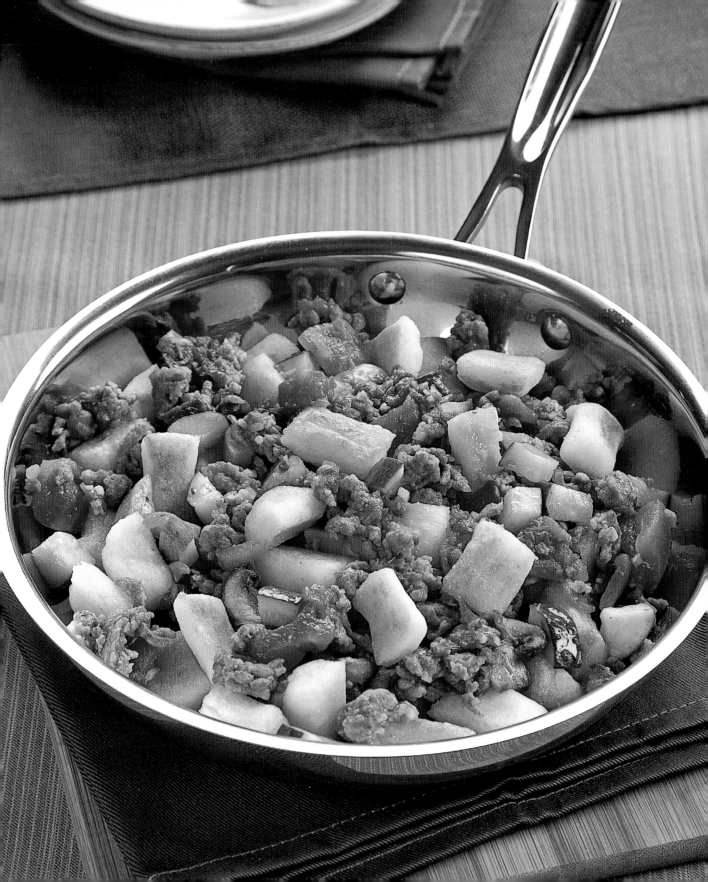

SUNDAY BRISKET

Makes 8 servings

       2 medium onions, thinly sliced
       1 small flat-cut boneless beef brisket (2 pounds), well trimmed
       1 cup gluten-free beef or chicken broth
       2 teaspoons dried thyme
       2 teaspoons paprika
       2 teaspoons garlic salt
       1 teaspoon black pepper
    1½ pounds unpeeled red potatoes, cut into 1-inch pieces
       1 pound baby carrots
       1 tablespoon cold water
       1 tablespoon cornstarch

1. Preheat oven to 350°F. Arrange onion rings in roasting pan. Place brisket over onions. Drizzle broth over brisket. Combine thyme, paprika, garlic salt and pepper in small bowl; sprinkle half of mixture over brisket. Turn brisket over; sprinkle with remaining mixture. Roast, covered, 2 hours and 25 minutes.

2. Remove brisket from oven; arrange potatoes and carrots around brisket in pan juices. Roast, covered, 45 minutes to 1 hour or until brisket is fork-tender and vegetables are tender.

3. Transfer brisket to cutting board; tent loosely with foil and let stand 15 minutes.

4. Transfer vegetables to serving bowl using slotted spoon; cover and keep warm. Pour pan juices into medium saucepan; spoon off and discard any fat. Stir water into cornstarch in small bowl until smooth. Stir into pan juices; simmer about 5 minutes or until thickened.

5. Carve brisket crosswise into thin slices; serve with vegetables and gravy.

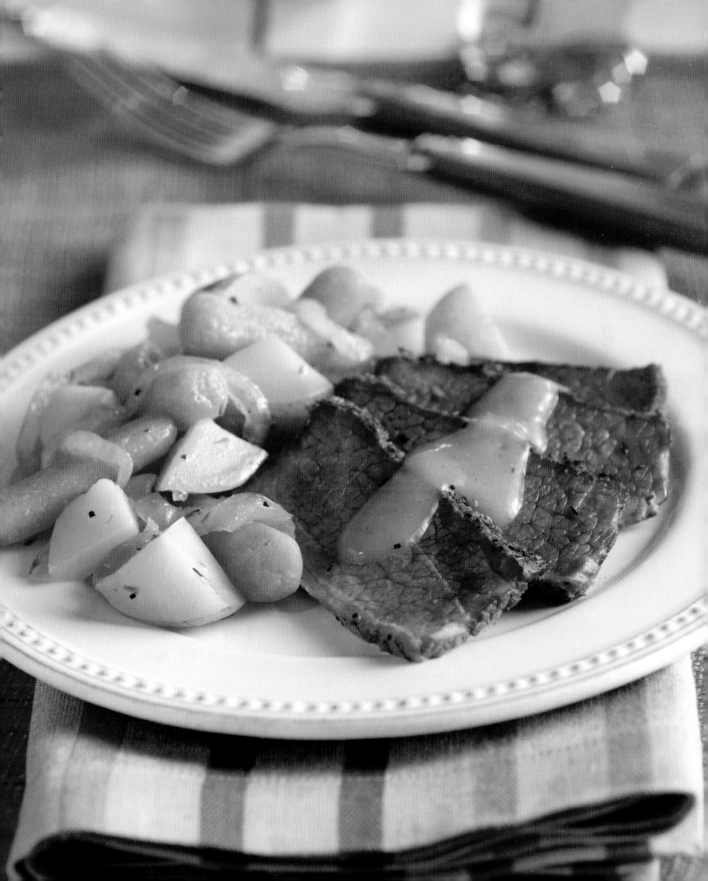

FISH AND "CHIPS"

Makes 4 servings

    3 cups gluten-free crisp rice cereal, divided
    1 egg
    1 tablespoon water
    1 pound cod, haddock or other firm white fish fillets, cut into 2×4-inch strips
    1½ teaspoons Italian seasoning, divided
       Salt and black pepper
    3 tablespoons butter, melted and divided
    2 medium zucchini, cut into sticks
    1 package (8 ounces) carrot sticks

1. Preheat oven to 350°F. Spray large baking sheet with nonstick cooking spray or line with foil.

2. Place 2 cups cereal in resealable food storage bag; coarsely crush with rolling pin. Combine with remaining 1 cup cereal in large shallow dish. Beat egg and water in separate shallow dish.

3. Sprinkle fish with 1 teaspoon Italian seasoning and season with salt and pepper. Dip in egg, letting excess drip back into dish. Coat in cereal, pressing lightly to adhere. Place on prepared baking sheet. Drizzle with 2 tablespoons butter.

4. Place zucchini and carrot sticks in single layer on same baking sheet. Drizzle with remaining 1 tablespoon butter and sprinkle with remaining ½ teaspoon Italian seasoning. Season with salt and pepper.

5. Bake 20 to 25 minutes or until fish is opaque in center and flakes easily when tested with fork.

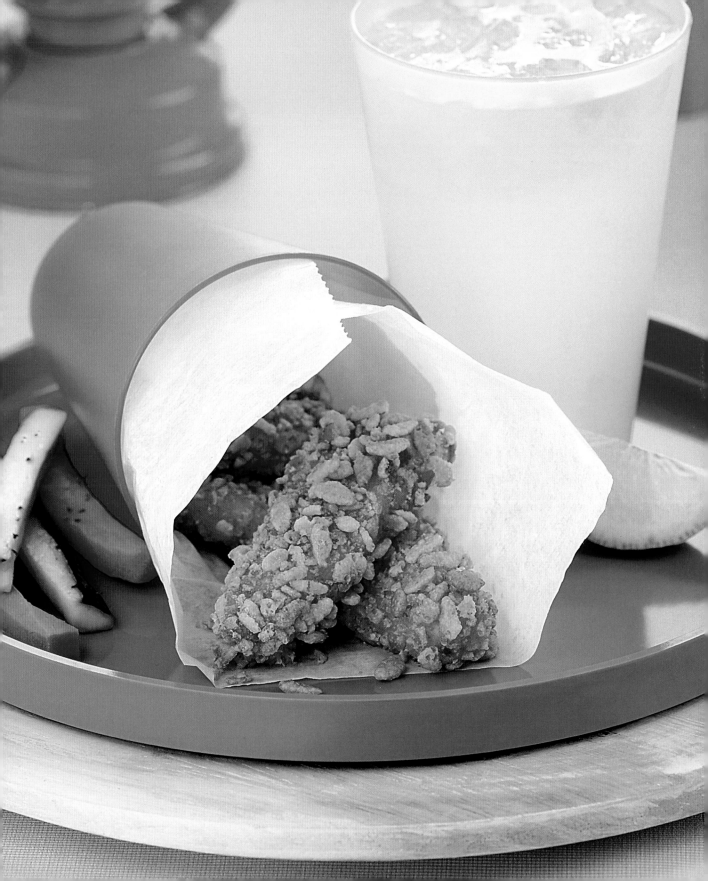

BAKED HAM WITH SWEET AND SPICY GLAZE

Makes 8 to 10 servings

> 1 (8-pound) bone-in smoked half ham
> Sweet and Spicy Glaze (recipe follows)

1. Preheat oven to 325°F. Place ham, fat side up, in roasting pan. Bake 3 hours.

2. Prepare Sweet and Spicy Glaze. Remove ham from oven. Generously brush half of glaze over ham; bake 30 minutes or until thermometer inserted into thickest part of ham registers 160°F.

3. Remove ham from oven; brush with remaining glaze. Let stand about 20 minutes before slicing.

SWEET AND SPICY GLAZE

Makes about 2 cups

> ¾ cup packed brown sugar
> ⅓ cup cider vinegar
> ¼ cup golden raisins
> 1 can (8¾ ounces) sliced peaches in heavy syrup, drained, chopped and syrup
>   reserved
> 1 tablespoon cornstarch
> ¼ cup orange juice
> 1 can (8¼ ounces) crushed pineapple in syrup, undrained
> 1 tablespoon grated orange peel
> 1 clove garlic, minced
> ½ teaspoon red pepper flakes
> ½ teaspoon grated fresh ginger

1. Combine brown sugar, vinegar, raisins and peach syrup in medium saucepan. Bring to a boil over high heat. Reduce heat to low; simmer 8 to 10 minutes.

2. Whisk cornstarch into orange juice in small bowl until smooth and well blended. Stir into brown sugar mixture. Stir pineapple, orange peel, garlic, red pepper flakes and ginger into saucepan; bring to a boil over medium heat. Cook until sauce is thickened, stirring constantly.

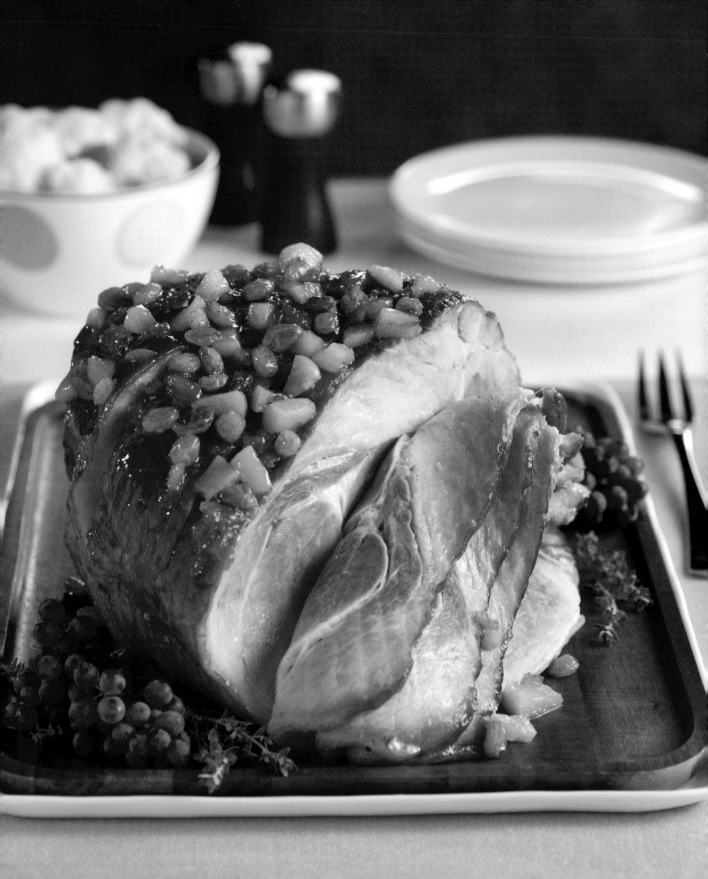

CREAMY CHEESE AND MACARONI

Makes 6 to 8 servings

1½ cups uncooked gluten-free elbow macaroni
1 cup chopped onion
1 cup chopped red or green bell pepper
¾ cup chopped celery
1 cup cottage cheese
1 cup (4 ounces) shredded Swiss cheese
2 ounces pasteurized process cheese product, cubed
½ cup whole milk
3 egg whites
3 tablespoons rice flour
1 tablespoon butter
¼ teaspoon black pepper
¼ teaspoon gluten-free hot pepper sauce

1. Preheat oven to 350°F. Spray 2-quart casserole with nonstick cooking spray.

2. Prepare macaroni according to package directions. Add onion, bell pepper and celery during last 5 minutes of cooking. Drain macaroni and vegetables.

3. Combine cottage cheese, Swiss cheese, cheese product, milk, egg whites, rice flour, butter, black pepper and hot pepper sauce in food processor or blender; process until smooth. Stir cheese mixture into macaroni and vegetables. Pour mixture into prepared casserole.

4. Bake 35 to 40 minutes or until golden brown. Let stand 10 minutes before serving.

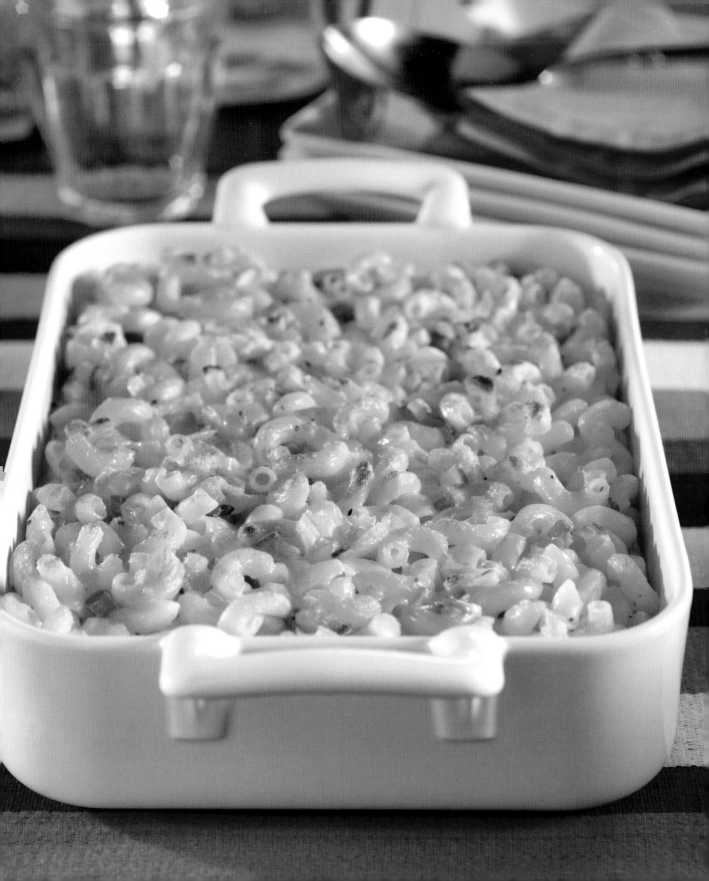

BEEF STEW STROGANOFF

Makes 6 servings

   2 tablespoons olive or canola oil
1½ pounds lean boneless beef (bottom round), cut into 1-inch cubes
   1 teaspoon caraway seeds
  ½ teaspoon salt
  ½ teaspoon black pepper
  ½ teaspoon dried thyme
   2 cans (about 14 ounces each) gluten-free beef broth
   1 cup sliced mushrooms
  ½ cup thinly sliced carrots
  ½ cup chopped red bell pepper
   6 ounces unpeeled baby red potatoes (about 6 small), quartered
  ¼ cup sour cream

1. Heat oil in large saucepan over medium-high heat. Add beef; cook and stir until meat juices evaporate and begin to caramelize. Add caraway seeds, salt, black pepper and thyme. Pour in broth, stirring to scrape up browned bits. Bring to a boil.

2. Add mushrooms, carrots and bell pepper to saucepan. Reduce heat; cover and simmer 1 hour.

3. Increase heat; add potatoes. Bring to a boil. Reduce heat; cover and simmer 20 minutes.

4. Stir in sour cream; cook 2 minutes or until heated through.

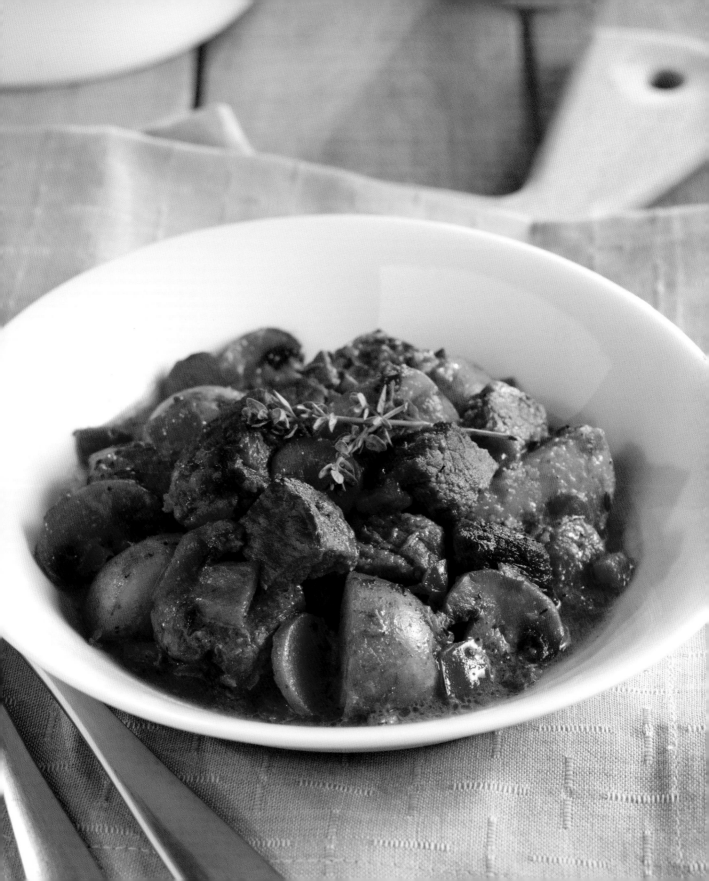

Sweet Treats

BEST EVER APPLE CRISP

Makes 8 servings

    8 cups thinly sliced peeled tart apples
    1 cup packed brown sugar, divided
    1 tablespoon cornstarch
    1½ teaspoons ground cinnamon, divided
    ¼ cup Gluten-Free All-Purpose Flour Blend (page 19)*
    ¼ cup (½ stick) cold unsalted butter, cubed
    ¾ cup gluten-free old-fashioned oats
    ½ cup coarsely chopped pecans
       Vanilla ice cream (optional)

Or use any all-purpose gluten-free flour blend that does not contain xanthan gum.

1. Preheat oven to 350°F.

2. Combine apples, ½ cup brown sugar, cornstarch and 1 teaspoon cinnamon in large bowl; toss to coat evenly. Spoon into 2-quart casserole.

3. Combine remaining ½ cup brown sugar, flour blend and remaining ½ teaspoon cinnamon in medium bowl; mix well. Cut in butter with pastry blender or two knives until coarse crumbs form. Stir in oats and pecans. Sprinkle evenly over apples.

4. Bake 40 to 45 minutes or until apples are tender and topping is brown. Serve warm with ice cream, if desired.

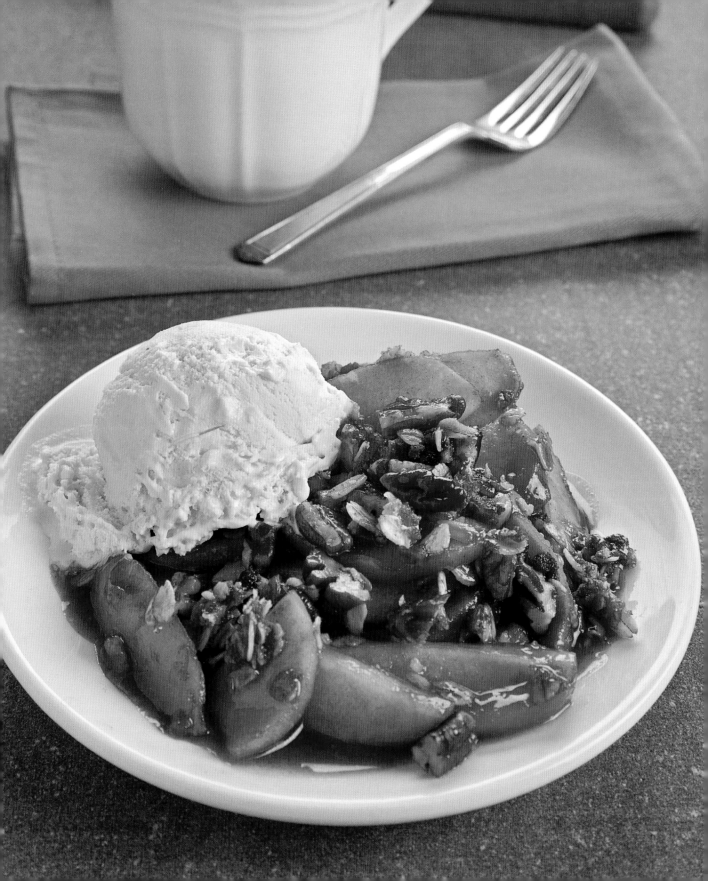

CHOCOLATE MARBLE & PRALINE CHEESECAKE

Makes 12 to 16 servings

Crust

   2 cups gluten-free shortbread cookie crumbs
   ½ cup finely chopped toasted pecans*
   6 tablespoons (¾ stick) butter, melted
   ¼ cup powdered sugar

Cheesecake

   3 packages (8 ounces each) cream cheese, softened
   1¼ cups packed brown sugar
   3 eggs, lightly beaten
   ½ cup sour cream
   1½ teaspoons vanilla
   1 square (1 ounce) unsweetened chocolate, melted
   20 to 25 pecan halves (½ cup)
   Gluten-free caramel ice cream topping

*To toast pecans, spread in a single layer on ungreased baking sheet. Bake in preheated 350°F oven 8 to 10 minutes or until fragrant, stirring occasionally.

1. Preheat oven to 350°F.

2. Combine cookie crumbs, chopped pecans, butter and powdered sugar in food processor; pulse until combined. Press onto bottom and up side of ungreased 9-inch springform pan. Bake 10 to 15 minutes or until lightly browned. Cool completely on wire rack.

3. Beat cream cheese in large bowl with electric mixer at medium speed until fluffy. Beat in brown sugar until smooth. Add eggs, sour cream and vanilla; beat just until blended. Remove 1 cup batter to small bowl; stir in chocolate.

4. Pour plain batter into prepared crust. Drop spoonfuls of chocolate batter over plain batter. Run knife through batters to marbleize. Arrange pecan halves around edge.

5. Bake 50 minutes or until set. Cool completely in pan on wire rack. Cover and refrigerate 2 hours or until ready to serve. Drizzle with topping.

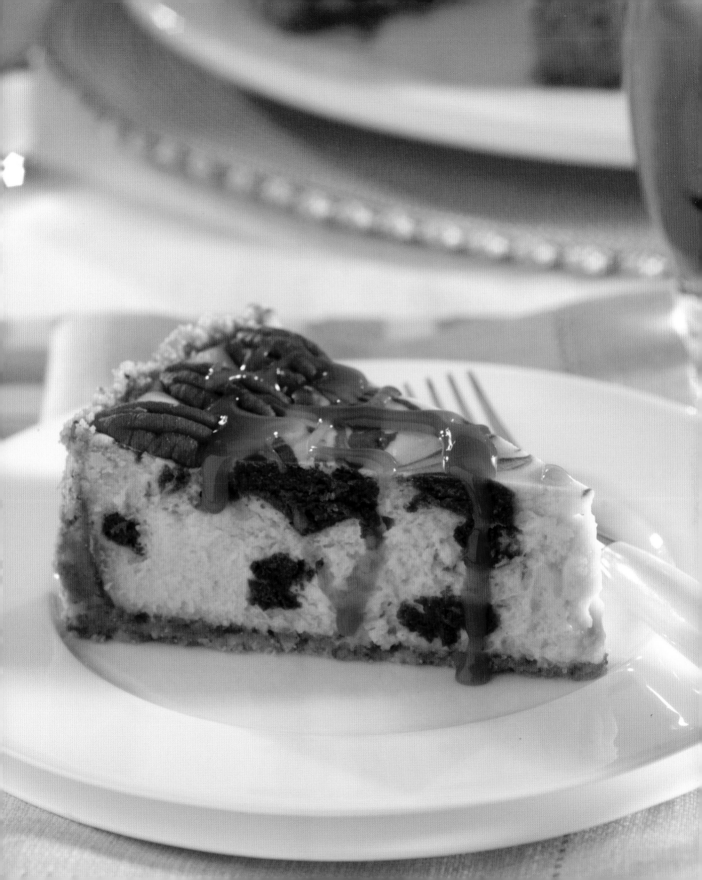

THUMBPRINT COOKIES

Makes 2 dozen cookies

   1 cup (2 sticks) butter, softened
   ½ cup packed dark brown sugar
   2 egg yolks
   2 teaspoons vanilla
   2 cups Gluten-Free All-Purpose Flour Blend (page 19)*
   ½ teaspoon salt
   2 egg whites, lightly beaten
 2¼ cups chopped walnuts
   ¼ cup raspberry jam

*Or use any all-purpose gluten-free flour blend that does not contain xanthan gum.

1. Preheat oven to 375°F. Line cookie sheets with parchment paper.

2. Beat butter and brown sugar in large bowl with electric mixer at medium-high speed 2 minutes or until light and fluffy. Add egg yolks and vanilla; beat at low speed, scraping side of bowl occasionally. Beat in flour blend and salt just until combined.

3. Place egg whites in shallow dish. Place walnuts in separate shallow dish. Roll tablespoons of dough into balls; dip in egg whites and roll in walnuts. Place on prepared cookie sheets.

4. Using thumb or back of small spoon, make small indentation in center of each ball; fill with jam.

5. Bake 12 to 15 minutes or until golden brown and filling is set, rotating cookie sheets halfway through baking time. Cool on cookie sheets 5 minutes. Remove to wire racks; cool completely.

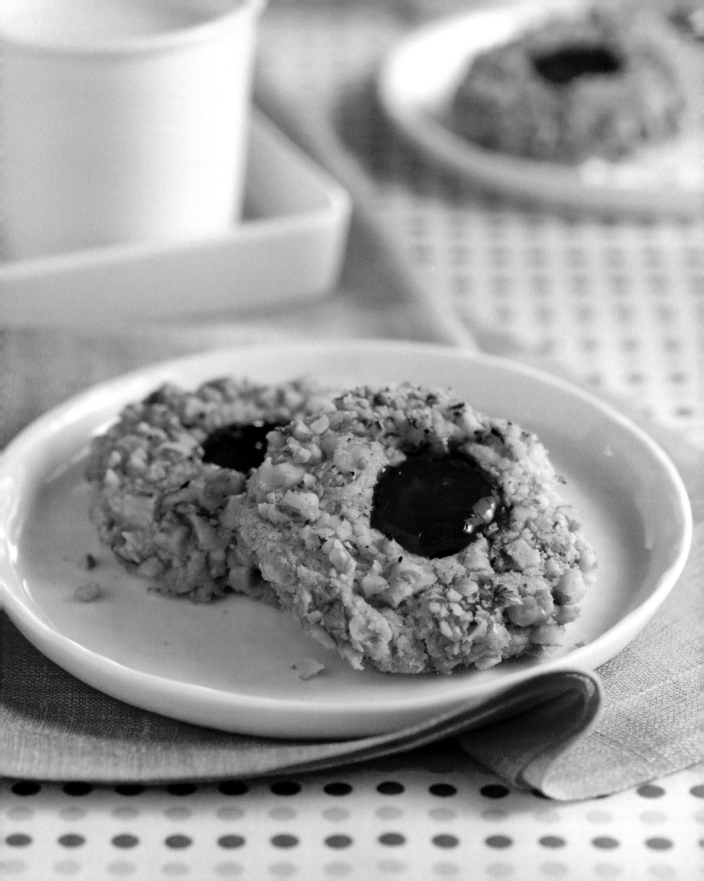

PUMPKIN-PINEAPPLE PIE

Makes 8 servings

   Gluten-Free Graham Cracker Crust (recipe follows)
1 can (8 ounces) pineapple rings in juice, undrained
2 tablespoons powdered egg replacer
1 can (15 ounces) solid-pack pumpkin
1 can (14 ounces) sweetened condensed milk
1 teaspoon ground cinnamon
1 teaspoon ground nutmeg
½ teaspoon ground ginger
⅛ teaspoon salt
1 tablespoon butter
   Whipped cream and fresh mint leaves (optional)

1. Preheat oven to 350°F. Prepare Gluten-Free Graham Cracker Crust. Drain pineapple; reserve ¼ cup juice. Set aside 4 pineapple rings; reserve remaining pineapple for another use.

2. Beat egg replacer and ¼ cup reserved pineapple juice in medium bowl with electric mixer at low speed until smooth. Add pumpkin, condensed milk, cinnamon, nutmeg, ginger and salt; beat until fluffy. Pour into prepared crust

3. Bake 45 to 50 minutes or until center is set. Cool completely in pan on wire rack.

4. Meanwhile, melt butter in small skillet over medium heat. Add pineapple rings; cook and stir until lightly golden. Cool completely.

5. To serve, arrange pineapple rings on top of pie; top with whipped cream, if desired. Garnish with mint.

GLUTEN-FREE GRAHAM CRACKER CRUST

Makes 1 (10-inch) deep-dish pie crust

25 gluten-free graham crackers, broken into small pieces
¾ cup (1½ sticks) butter, cubed
⅓ cup sugar

1. Preheat oven to 350°F. Grease 10-inch deep-dish pie pan.

2. Place graham crackers in food processor; pulse until finely crushed. Add butter and sugar; process until well combined. Press mixture firmly onto bottom and up side of prepared pan.

3. Bake 8 minutes or until browned. Cool completely.

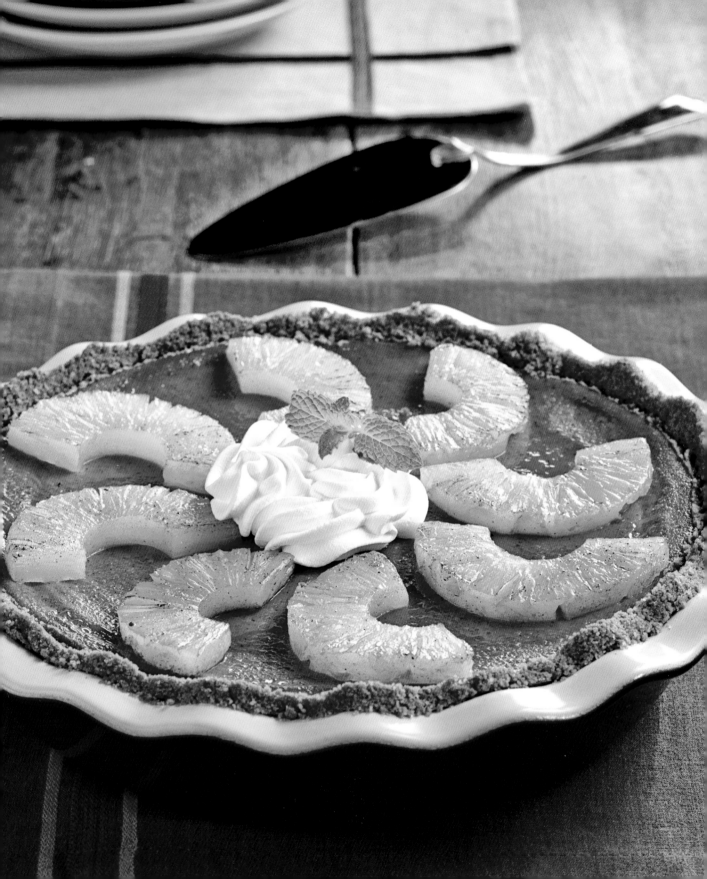

WHITE CHOCOLATE PUDDING WITH CRUNCHY TOFFEE TOPPING

Makes 6 servings

  ¼ cup sugar
  ¼ cup cornstarch *or* 1¾ teaspoons guar gum
  ¼ teaspoon salt
   2 cups milk
  ¾ cup whipping cream
   7 squares (1 ounce each) white chocolate, chopped
   2 teaspoons vanilla
     Crunchy Toffee Topping (recipe follows)

1. Combine sugar, cornstarch and salt in medium saucepan; mix well. Slowly whisk in milk and cream. Bring to a boil over medium heat, stirring constantly. Reduce heat; cook and stir 2 to 3 minutes or until mixture is thickened.

2. Remove from heat; stir in white chocolate and vanilla until white chocolate is completely melted. Spoon into six dessert dishes; cover with plastic wrap. Refrigerate 1 hour or up to 2 days.

3. Prepare Crunchy Toffee Topping. Sprinkle over pudding just before serving.

CRUNCHY TOFFEE TOPPING

  ½ cup sugar
  ¼ cup light corn syrup
   1 cup sliced almonds
   2 teaspoons butter
  ½ teaspoon baking soda
  ½ teaspoon vanilla

1. Spray 10-inch square sheet of foil with nonstick cooking spray.

2. Whisk sugar and corn syrup in small microwavable bowl. Microwave on HIGH 4 minutes. (Mixture will be light brown in color.) Stir in almonds and butter; microwave on HIGH 2 minutes. Stir in baking soda and vanilla. (Mixture will foam.)

3. Spread mixture in thin layer on prepared foil; cool completely. Break into pieces.

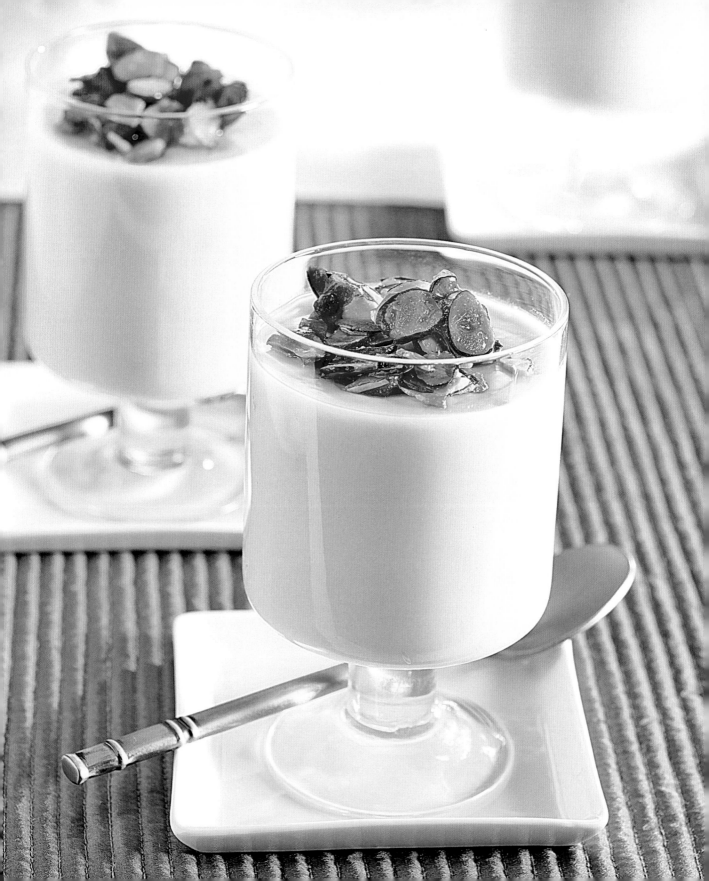

OLD-FASHIONED BREAD PUDDING

Makes 6 to 8 servings

   10 slices gluten-free cinnamon-raisin bread, cut into ½-inch cubes
   ¼ cup (½ stick) butter, melted
   2 cups whole milk
   4 eggs
   ¾ cup sugar
   2 teaspoons ground cinnamon
   1 teaspoon vanilla
   ½ cup raisins
   ½ cup chopped dried apples

1. Grease 9-inch baking dish.

2. Combine bread cubes and butter in prepared baking dish; toss to coat.

3. Whisk milk, eggs, sugar, cinnamon and vanilla in medium bowl. Stir in raisins and dried apples. Pour over bread cubes. Cover and refrigerate at least 2 hours.

4. Preheat oven to 350°F. Bake 50 to 55 minutes or until golden brown and center is set. Let stand 10 minutes before serving.

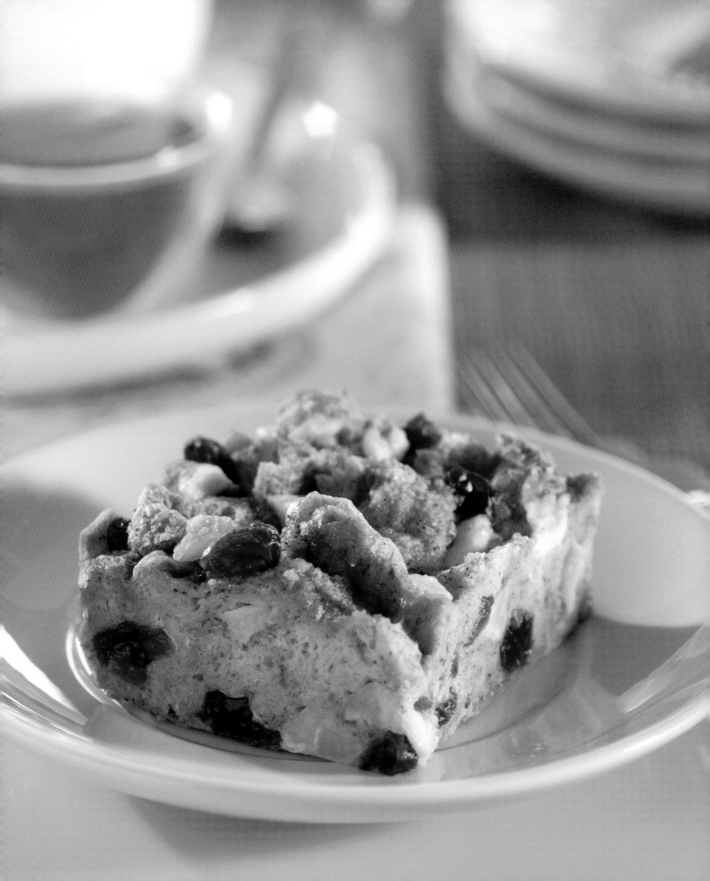

PECAN PIE

Makes 8 servings

>   **Gluten-Free Pie Crust (recipe follows)**
> **3 eggs**
> **¾ cup dark corn syrup**
> **¾ cup sugar**
> **1 teaspoon vanilla**
> **¼ teaspoon salt**
> **2 cups chopped pecans**

1. Prepare Gluten-Free Pie Crust. Preheat oven to 425°F. Lightly grease 9-inch pie pan. Place pie crust in prepared pan. Flute edge as desired.

2. Beat eggs in large bowl. Add corn syrup, sugar, vanilla and salt; beat until well blended. Pour over crust; sprinkle evenly with pecans.

3. Bake 45 to 50 minutes or until set. Cool completely in pan on wire rack.

Tip: If edges brown too quickly in oven, cover with a strip of foil.

GLUTEN-FREE PIE CRUST

Makes 1 (9- to 10-inch) pie crust

>   **1 cup Gluten-Free All-Purpose Flour Blend (page 19),* plus additional for work surface**
> **2 tablespoons sweet rice flour (mochiko)**
> **1½ teaspoons sugar**
> **½ teaspoon xanthan gum**
> **¼ teaspoon salt**
> **6 tablespoons (¾ stick) cold butter, cubed**
> **1 egg**
> **2 teaspoons cider vinegar**

*Or use any all-purpose gluten-free flour blend that does not contain xanthan gum.

1. Combine 1 cup flour blend, sweet rice flour, sugar, xanthan gum and salt in medium bowl; mix well. Cut in butter with pastry blender or two knives until coarse crumbs form.

2. Make well in center of mixture. Add egg and vinegar and stir just until dough forms. Shape dough into flat disc. Wrap in plastic wrap and refrigerate at least 45 minutes or until very cold.

3. Roll out dough on floured surface into circle slightly larger than pie plate. (If dough becomes sticky, refrigerate until cold.) Wrap in plastic wrap and refrigerate until ready to use.

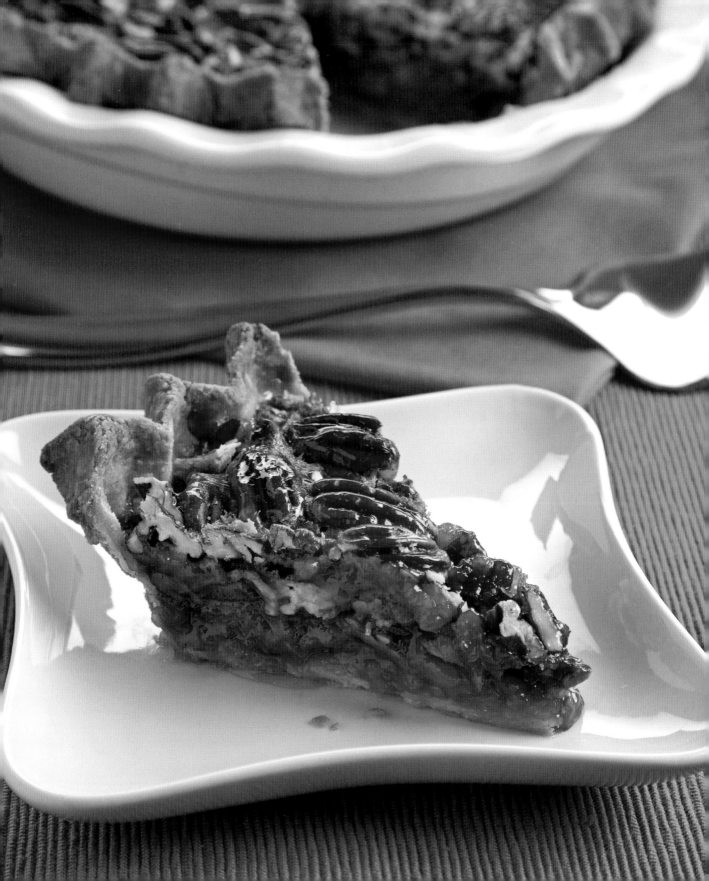

CHERRY CHEESECAKE SWIRL BARS

Makes 16 servings

Crust

1⅔ cups gluten-free shortbread cookie crumbs
½ cup (1 stick) butter, melted
¼ cup sugar

Cheesecake

2 packages (8 ounces each) cream cheese, softened
½ cup sugar
3 eggs
½ cup sour cream
½ teaspoon almond extract
3 tablespoons cherry preserves, melted and strained

1. Preheat oven to 325°F.

2. Combine cookie crumbs, butter and ¼ cup sugar in medium bowl; mix well. Press crumb mixture onto bottom of 9-inch square baking pan. Bake 10 minutes or until set but not browned. Cool completely.

3. Beat cream cheese in medium bowl with electric mixer at medium speed until fluffy. Add ½ cup sugar; beat until smooth. Add eggs, one at a time, beating well after each addition. Add sour cream and almond extract; beat until well blended. Spread evenly in prepared crust.

4. Drizzle melted preserves in zigzag pattern over cheesecake batter. Drag tip of knife through jam and batter to make swirls.

5. Place pan in 13×9-inch baking dish; add water to come halfway up sides of cheesecake.

6. Bake 45 to 50 minutes or until knife inserted 1 inch from edge comes out clean. Cool completely in pan on wire rack. Cover and refrigerate 2 hours or until ready to serve.

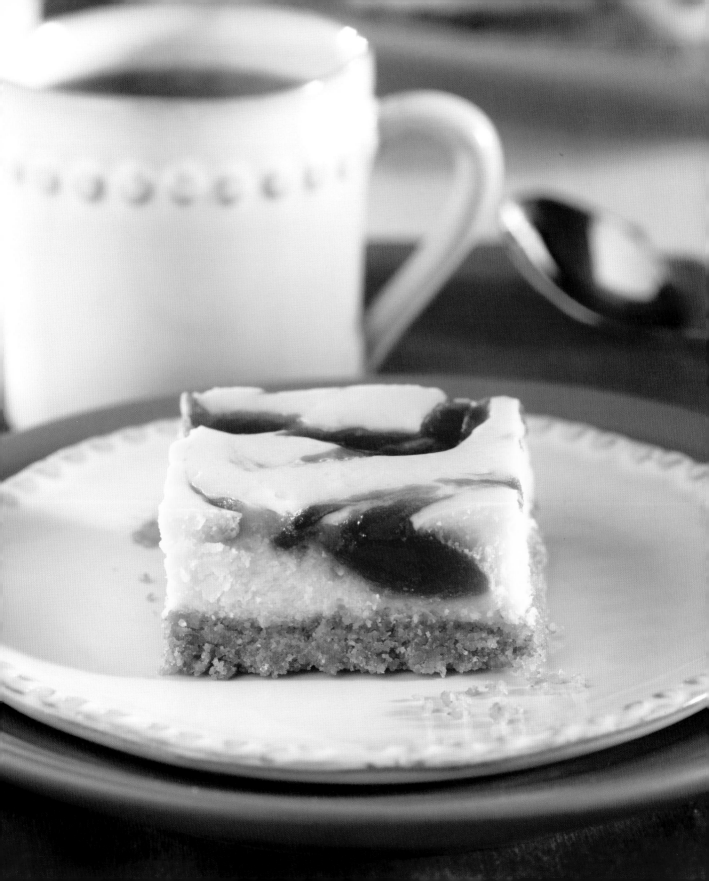

CRANBERRY PEAR COBBLER

Makes 8 servings

Filling

    3 pounds ripe pears (6 pears), peeled and sliced
  1½ cups cranberries
   ¼ cup granulated sugar
   1 tablespoon cornstarch
   1 tablespoon grated orange peel
   1 teaspoon ground cinnamon

Topping

   1 package (about 15 ounces) gluten-free yellow cake mix
   1 cup low-fat buttermilk
   ½ cup (1 stick) butter, softened
   2 teaspoons vanilla
  1½ tablespoons packed brown sugar
  1½ tablespoons granulated sugar
    Whipped cream (optional)

1. Preheat oven to 400°F. Spray 13×9-inch baking dish with nonstick cooking spray.

2. Combine pears, cranberries, ¼ cup granulated sugar, cornstarch, orange peel and cinnamon in large bowl; toss to coat. Pour into prepared baking dish.

3. Bake 20 minutes or until bubbly.

4. Meanwhile, beat cake mix, buttermilk, butter and vanilla in large bowl with electric mixer at low speed 30 seconds or until moistened. Beat at medium speed 2 minutes.

5. Remove baking dish from oven. Pour topping evenly over filling. Sprinkle with brown sugar and 1½ tablespoons granulated sugar.

6. Bake 30 to 35 minutes or until topping is golden brown. Serve warm with whipped cream, if desired.

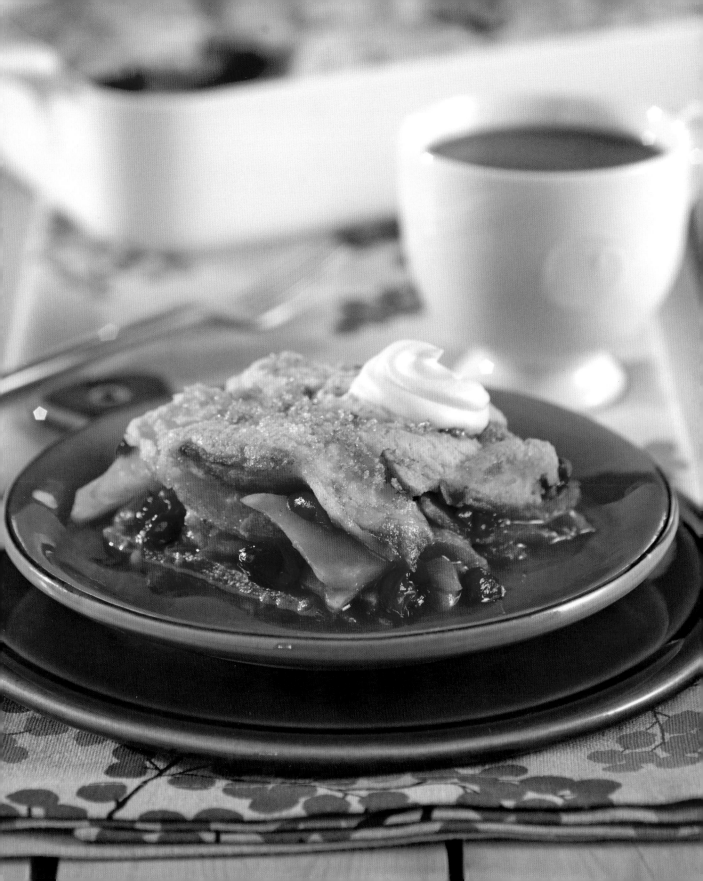

CLASSIC BROWNIES

Makes 9 brownies

¼ cup soy flour
¼ cup cornstarch
½ teaspoon baking soda
¼ teaspoon salt
½ cup (1 stick) butter
1 cup packed brown sugar
½ cup unsweetened cocoa powder
½ cup semisweet chocolate chips
1 teaspoon vanilla
2 eggs

1. Preheat oven to 350°F. Spray 8-inch square baking pan with nonstick cooking spray.

2. Combine soy flour, cornstarch, baking soda and salt in small bowl; mix well

3. Melt butter in large saucepan over low heat. Add brown sugar; cook and stir until sugar is dissolved. Remove from heat; sift in cocoa and stir until combined. Stir in flour mixture until smooth. (Mixture will be thick.)

4. Stir in chocolate chips and vanilla. Add eggs; beat until smooth and well blended. Pour into prepared pan.

5. Bake 25 to 30 minutes or until toothpick inserted into center comes out almost clean.

TIP

This basic recipe can be made with a twist. Try substituting other gluten-free baking chips for the chocolate, like white chocolate.

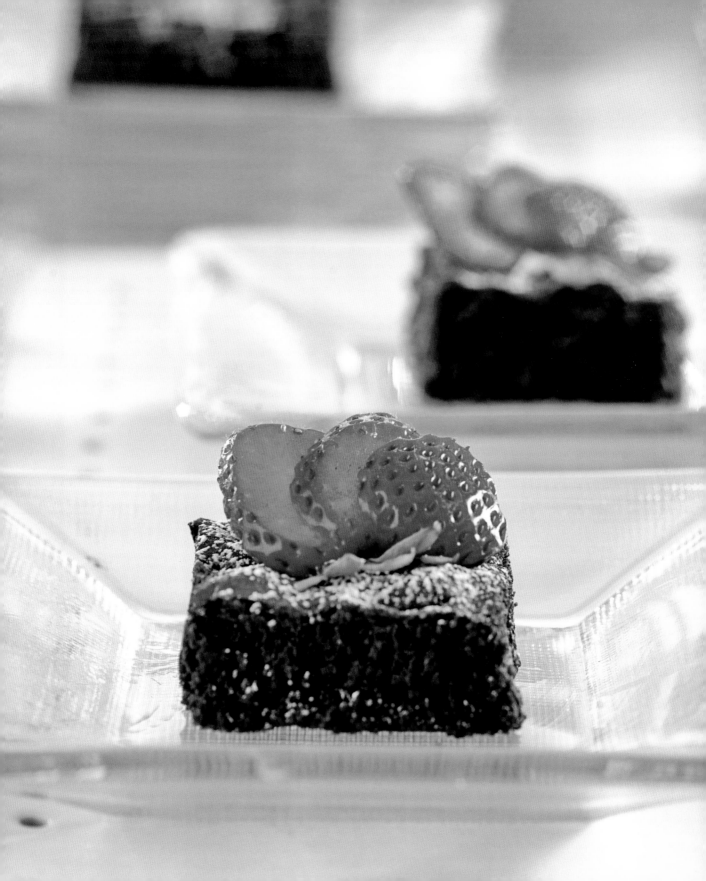

BANANA-COCONUT CREAM PIE

Makes 8 servings

Crust

>   1 cup almonds
>   1 tablespoon sugar
>   ½ cup flaked coconut
>   ¼ cup (½ stick) butter, cut into pieces
>   ⅛ teaspoon salt

Filling

>   2 bananas
>   1 teaspoon lemon juice
>   ½ cup sugar
>   ¼ cup cornstarch
>   ¼ teaspoon salt
>   3 cups whole milk
>   2 egg yolks
>   1 teaspoon vanilla

Topping

>   1 banana
>   2 tablespoons flaked coconut, toasted*
>   Whipped cream

To toast coconut, spread in single layer in heavy-bottomed skillet. Cook over medium heat 1 to 2 minutes, stirring frequently, until lightly browned. Remove from skillet immediately. Cool before using.

1. Preheat oven to 350°F. Grease 9-inch pie pan. Place almonds and 1 tablespoon sugar in food processor; pulse until almonds are ground. Add ½ cup coconut; pulse until combined. Add butter and ⅛ teaspoon salt; pulse until mixture begins to stick together. Press onto bottom and up side of prepared pan. Bake 10 to 12 minutes or until golden around edge. Cool completely.

2. Slice 2 bananas; sprinkle with lemon juice. Layer on bottom of prepared crust.

3. Combine ½ cup sugar, cornstarch and ¼ teaspoon salt in medium saucepan. Whisk milk and egg yolks in medium bowl until well blended; slowly stir into sugar mixture. Cook and stir over medium heat until thickened. Bring to a boil; boil 1 minute. Remove from heat; stir in vanilla. Pour mixture over bananas in crust. Cover and refrigerate at least 2 hours.

4. Slice remaining banana; arrange on top of pie. Sprinkle with 2 tablespoons coconut and top with whipped cream.

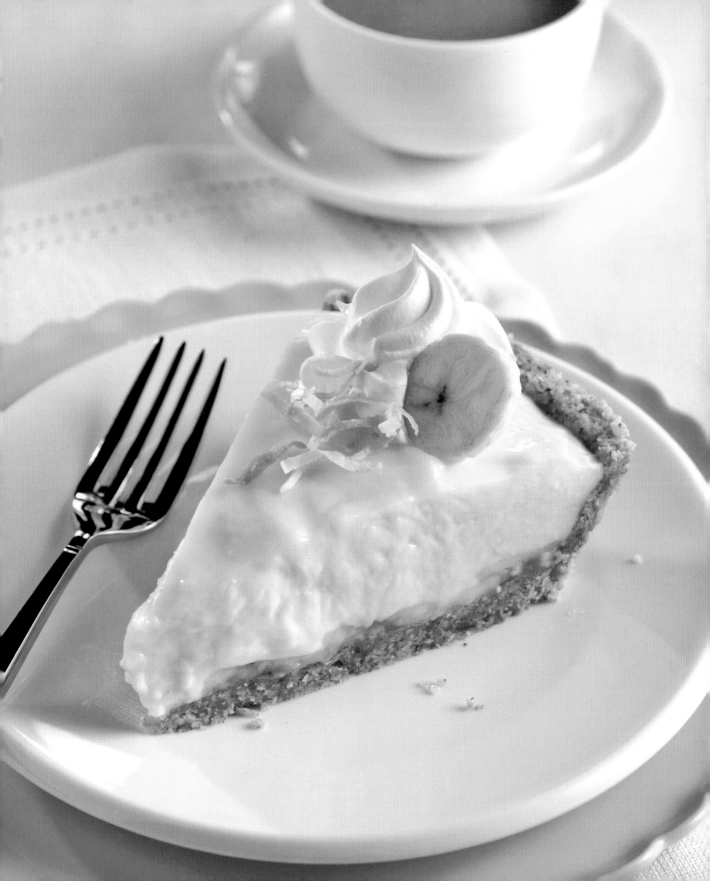

GINGERBREAD

Makes 9 servings

   2 cups Gluten-Free All-Purpose Flour Blend (page 19)*
   2 teaspoons ground ginger
   ¾ teaspoon xanthan gum
   ½ teaspoon baking powder
   ½ teaspoon baking soda
   ½ teaspoon salt
   ½ teaspoon ground cinnamon
   1 cup ginger ale
   ¾ cup packed brown sugar
   6 tablespoons (¾ stick) butter, melted and cooled
   ½ cup molasses
   2 eggs
   1 tablespoon grated fresh ginger
   Whipped cream (optional)

*Or use any all-purpose gluten-free flour blend that does not contain xanthan gum.

1. Preheat oven to 350°F. Spray 9-inch square baking pan with nonstick cooking spray.

2. Combine flour blend, ground ginger, xanthan gum, baking powder, baking soda, salt and cinnamon in medium bowl. Whisk ginger ale, brown sugar, butter, molasses, eggs and grated ginger in large bowl until well blended. Add flour mixture in two additions, stirring until well blended after each addition. Pour into prepared pan.

3. Bake 30 to 35 minutes or until toothpick inserted into center comes out clean. Cool in pan 10 minutes. Remove to wire rack to cool slightly. Serve warm or at room temperature with whipped cream, if desired.

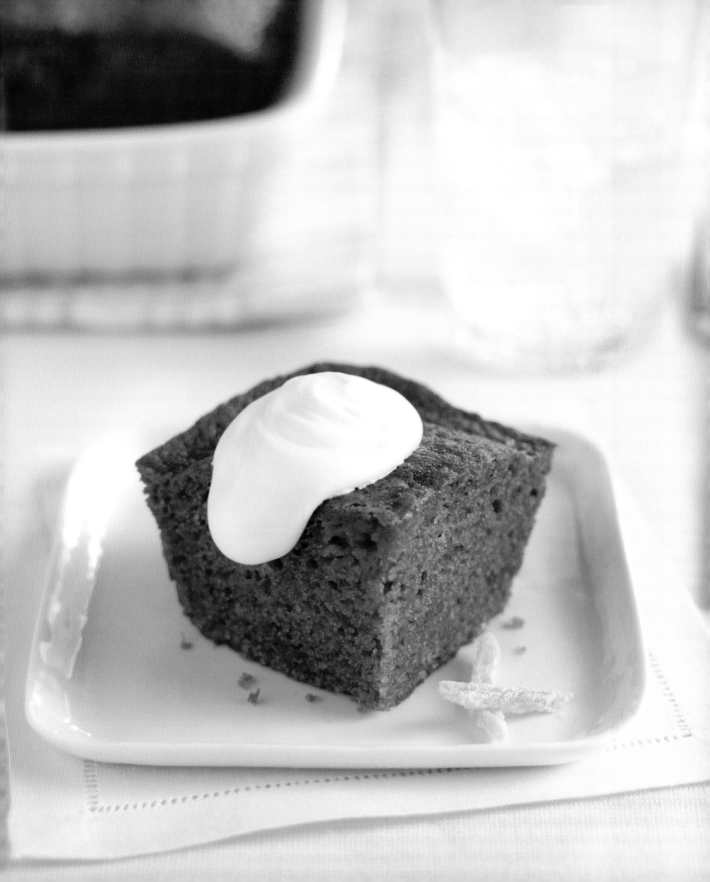

BUTTERSCOTCH TOFFEE GINGERSNAP SQUARES

Makes 3 dozen bars

    40 gluten-free gingersnap cookies
     6 tablespoons (¾ stick) butter, melted
     1 cup butterscotch chips*
    ½ cup pecan pieces
    ½ cup chopped peanuts
    ½ cup milk chocolate toffee bits
    ½ cup mini semisweet chocolate chips
     1 can (14 ounces) sweetened condensed milk
    1½ teaspoons vanilla

*Read labels carefully as not all butterscotch chips are gluten-free.

1. Preheat oven to 350°F. Line 13×9-inch baking pan with foil, leaving 1-inch overhang. Spray with nonstick cooking spray.

2. Place cookies in food processor; process until crumbs form. Measure 2 cups.

3. Combine 2 cups crumbs and butter in medium bowl; mix well. Press crumb mixture evenly onto bottom of prepared pan. Bake 4 to 5 minutes or until light brown around edges.

4. Meanwhile, combine butterscotch chips, pecans, peanuts, toffee bits and chocolate chips in medium bowl. Whisk condensed milk and vanilla in small bowl; pour over warm crust. Sprinkle with butterscotch mixture, pressing down gently.

5. Bake 15 to 18 minutes or until golden and bubbly. Cool completely in pan on wire rack. Remove foil; cut into bars.

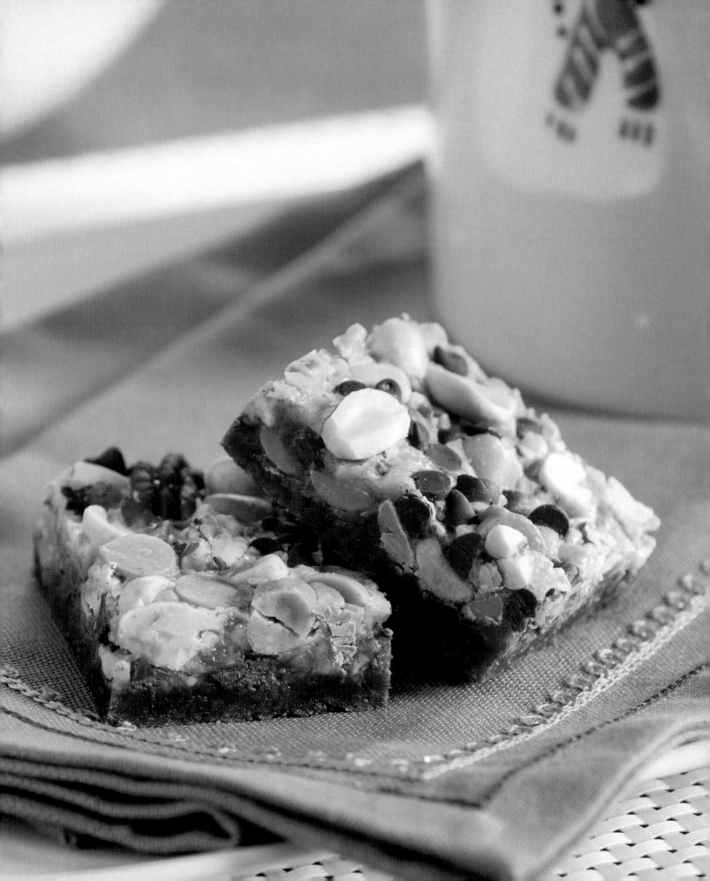

COCONUT-LEMON LAYER BARS

Makes about 32 bars

Crust

    1 cup gluten-free shortbread cookie crumbs

    ½ cup (1 stick) butter, melted

Filling

    1 package (8 ounces) cream cheese, softened

    Grated peel and juice of 1 lemon

    1 egg

    2 tablespoons sugar

    1 cup (6 ounces) white chocolate chips

    1 cup flaked coconut

    ½ cup chopped macadamia nuts

1. Preheat oven to 350°F. Spray 13×9-inch baking pan with nonstick cooking spray.

2. Combine cookie crumbs and butter in medium bowl; stir until well combined. Press crumb mixture onto bottom of prepared pan.

3. Beat cream cheese, lemon peel, lemon juice, egg and sugar in medium bowl with electric mixer at low speed until smooth. Spread evenly over crumb mixture.

4. Layer evenly with white chocolate chips, coconut and macadamia nuts, pressing down each layer firmly with fork.

5. Bake 25 to 30 minutes or until lightly browned. Cool completely. Cover and refrigerate until ready to serve.

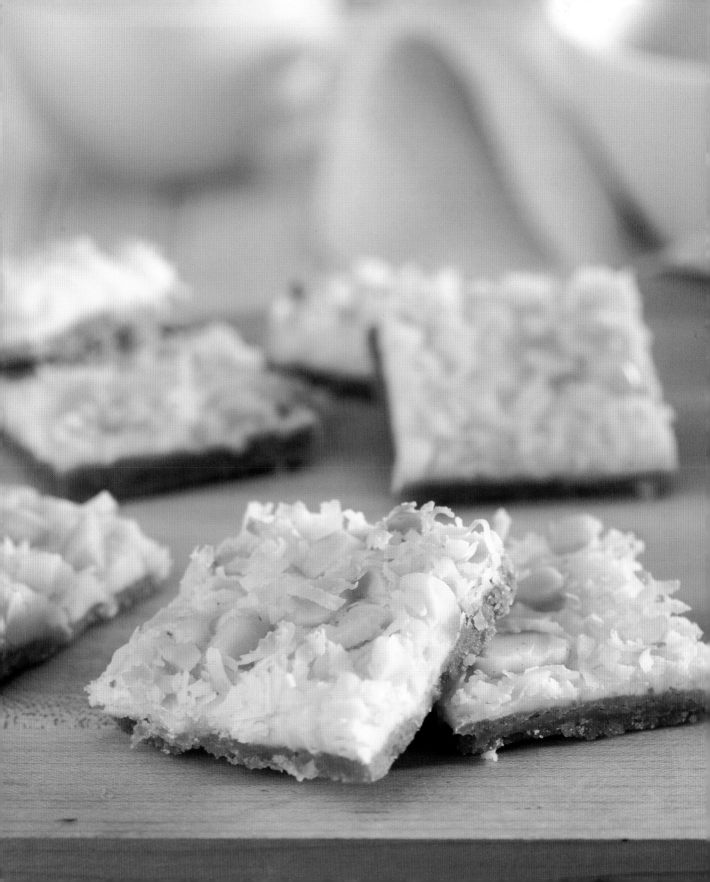

DARK CHOCOLATE RASPBERRY BREAD PUDDING

Makes 6 to 8 servings

    8 slices gluten-free white sandwich bread, cut into ½-inch cubes
    ¼ cup (½ stick) butter, melted
    2 cups whole milk
    4 eggs
    ¾ cup sugar
    1 teaspoon vanilla
    ½ cup raspberries
    ½ cup bittersweet or semisweet chocolate chips

1. Grease 9-inch baking dish.

2. Combine bread cubes and butter in prepared dish; toss to coat.

3. Whisk milk, eggs, sugar and vanilla in medium bowl. Pour over bread cubes. Cover and refrigerate 2 hours.

4. Preheat oven to 350°F. Sprinkle raspberries and chocolate chips evenly over bread mixture.

5. Bake 40 to 50 minutes or until golden brown and center is set. Let stand 10 minutes before serving.

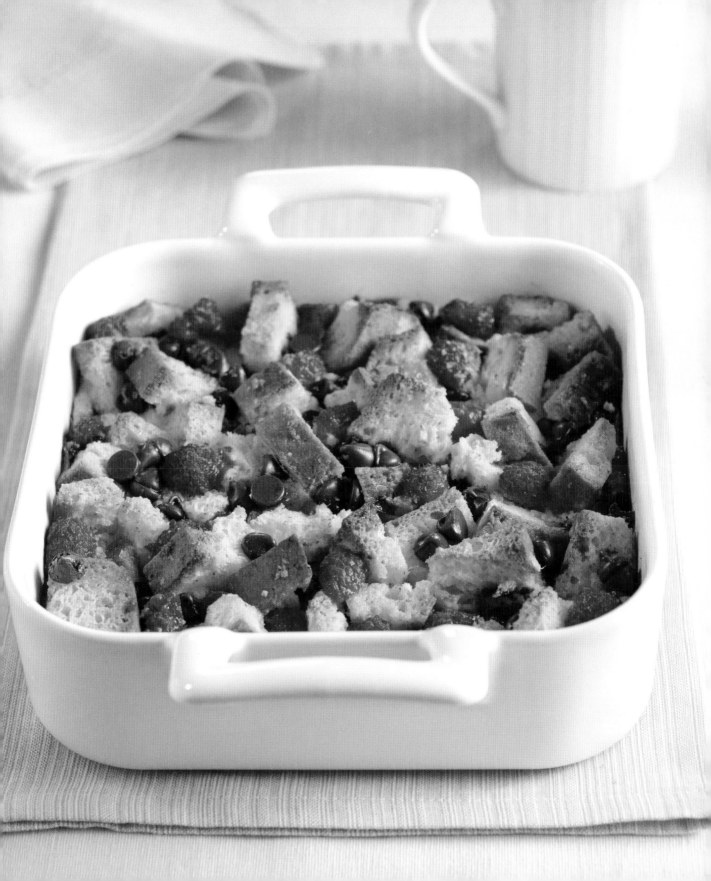

Snack Time

EDAMAME HUMMUS

Makes 2 cups (about 16 servings)

- 1 package (16 ounces) frozen shelled edamame, thawed
- ½ cup coarsely chopped green onions
- ½ cup loosely packed fresh cilantro
- 3 to 4 tablespoons water
- 2 tablespoons canola oil
- 1½ tablespoons fresh lime juice
- 1 tablespoon honey
- 2 cloves garlic
- 1 teaspoon salt
- ¼ teaspoon black pepper
- Rice crackers and/or vegetable sticks

1. Combine edamame, green onions, cilantro, 3 tablespoons water, oil, lime juice, honey, garlic, salt and pepper in food processor; process until smooth. Add additional water to thin dip, if necessary.

2. Serve with rice crackers and/or vegetable sticks for dipping. Store in refrigerator up to 4 days

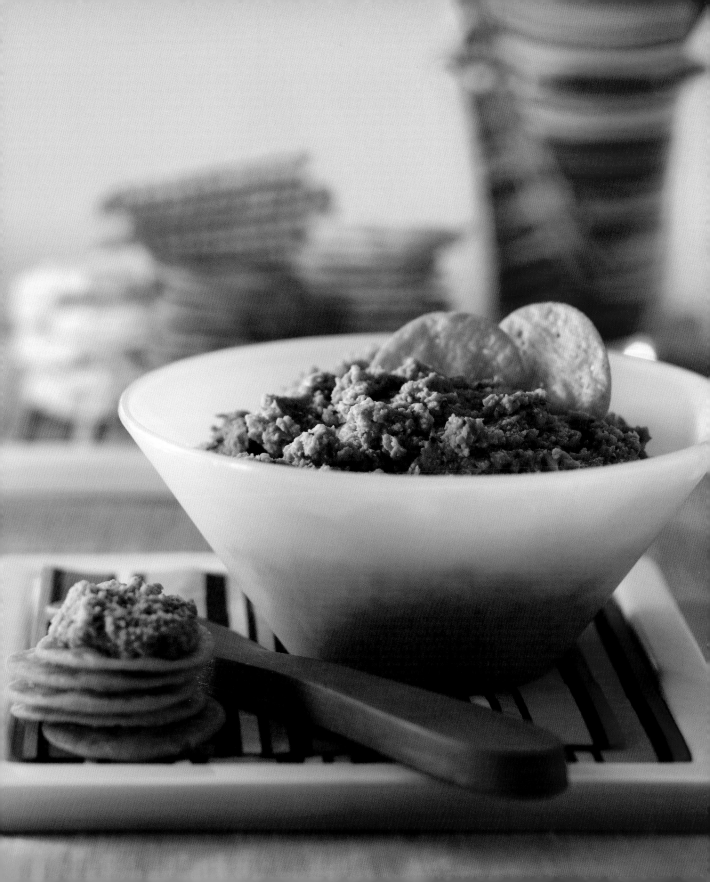

NO-BAKE FRUIT AND GRAIN BARS

Makes 16 bars

> ½ cup cooked amaranth
> 2 cups gluten-free whole grain puffed rice cereal
> ½ cup chopped dried fruit
> ½ cup honey
> ¼ cup sugar
> ¾ cup almond butter

1. Spray 8- or 9-inch square baking pan with nonstick cooking spray.

2. Heat medium saucepan over high heat. Add 1 tablespoon amaranth; stir or gently shake saucepan until almost all seeds have popped. (Partially cover saucepan if seeds are popping over the side.) Remove to medium bowl. Repeat with remaining amaranth.

3. Stir cereal and dried fruits into popped amaranth.

4. Combine honey and sugar in same saucepan; bring to a boil over medium heat. Remove from heat; stir in almond butter until melted and smooth.

5. Pour honey mixture over cereal mixture; stir until evenly coated. Press firmly into prepared pan. Let stand until set. Cut into bars

Note: Amaranth is a gluten-free whole grain that's high in protein and fiber. Cooked amaranth is tender with a slight crunch. It doesn't fluff up like rice, but instead has a dense quality that retains moisture.

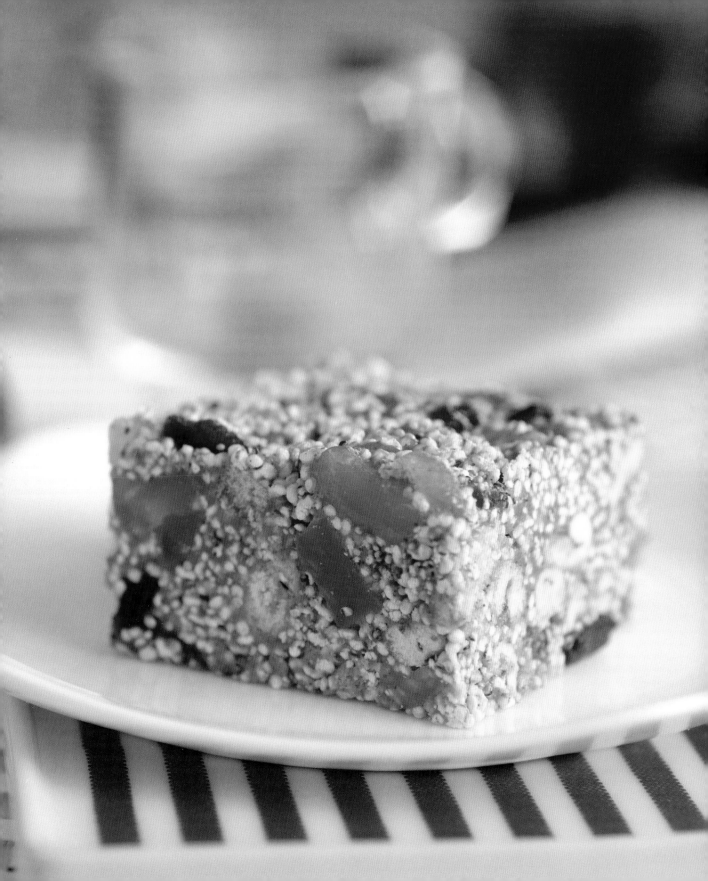

KALE CHIPS

Makes 6 servings

> 1 large bunch kale (about 1 pound)
> 1 to 2 tablespoons olive oil
> 1 teaspoon garlic salt or other seasoned salt

1. Preheat oven to 350°F. Line baking sheets with parchment paper.

2. Wash kale and pat dry with paper towels. Remove center ribs and stems; discard. Cut leaves into 2- to 3-inch-wide pieces.

3. Combine leaves, oil and garlic salt in large bowl; toss to coat. Spread on prepared baking sheets.

4. Bake 10 to 15 minutes or until edges are lightly browned and leaves are crisp.* Cool completely on baking sheets. Store in airtight container.

If the leaves are lightly browned but not crisp, turn oven off and let chips stand in oven until crisp, about 10 minutes. Do not keep the oven on as the chips will burn easily.

POLENTA PIZZAS

Makes 4 to 6 servings

> 1 teaspoon olive oil
> ½ cup chopped onion
> ¼ pound gluten-free bulk mild Italian sausage
> 1 can (8 ounces) gluten-free pizza sauce
> 1 roll (16 ounces) prepared polenta
> 1 cup (4 ounces) shredded mozzarella cheese

1. Preheat oven to 350°F. Spray 13×9-inch baking pan with nonstick cooking spray.

2. Heat oil in large nonstick skillet over medium heat. Add onion; cook and stir 3 minutes or until tender. Add sausage; cook 5 minutes or until browned, stirring to break up meat. Stir in pizza sauce; simmer 5 minutes.

3. Cut polenta roll into 16 slices; arrange in prepared pan. Spoon 1 heaping tablespoon sausage mixture and 1 tablespoon cheese over each polenta slice.

4. Bake 15 minutes or until heated through and cheese is melted.

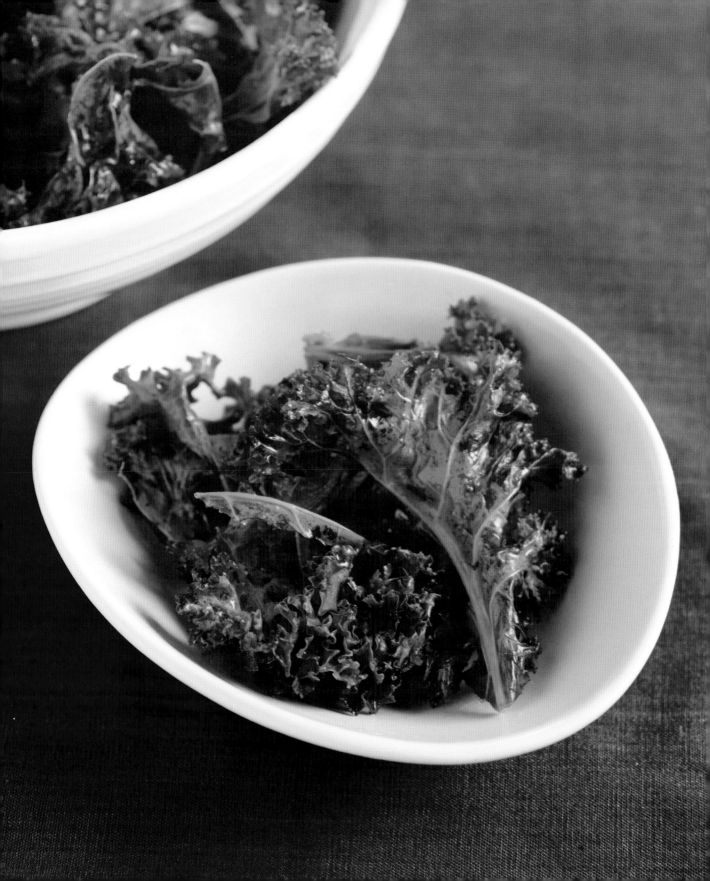

LEMONY ARROWROOT COOKIES

Makes 12 cookies

Cookies

   ¼ cup (½ stick) butter
   ⅓ cup granulated sugar
   1 egg
      Grated peel and juice of 1 lemon
   ½ teaspoon vanilla
   1¼ cups Gluten-Free All-Purpose Flour Blend (page 19),* plus additional for work surface
   ½ cup arrowroot
   ½ teaspoon baking powder
   ¼ teaspoon salt

Glaze

   ¼ cup powdered sugar
   1 teaspoon grated lemon peel, plus additional for garnish
   1 tablespoon lemon juice, plus additional if necessary

Or use any all-purpose gluten-free flour blend that does not contain xanthan gum.

1. Preheat oven to 350°F. Grease cookie sheet.

2. Beat butter and granulated sugar in large bowl with electric mixer at medium speed until creamy. Add egg, grated peel and juice of 1 lemon and vanilla; beat until well blended. Add 1¼ cups flour blend, arrowroot, baking powder and salt; beat at low speed just until combined.

3. Roll out dough onto floured surface to ⅛-inch thickness. Cut out shapes with desired cookie cutters. Place on prepared baking sheet.

4. Bake 8 to 10 minutes. (Cookies will not brown.) Remove to wire rack; cool completely.

5. Combine powdered sugar and 1 teaspoon lemon peel in small bowl; stir in enough lemon juice to make pourable glaze. Drizzle glaze over cookies. Garnish with additional lemon peel.

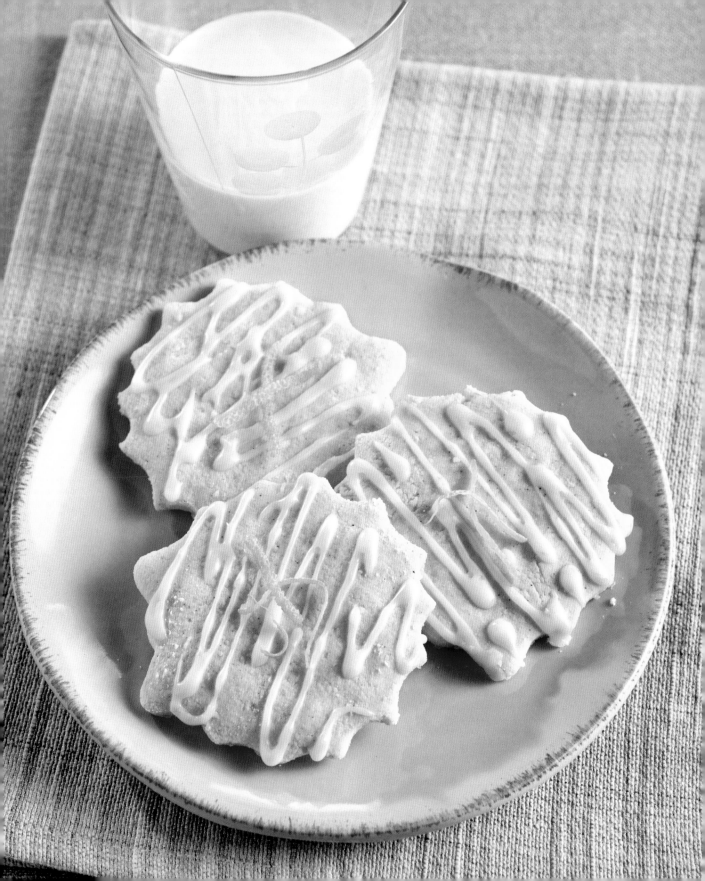

DOUBLE BERRY POPS

Makes 6 pops

> **2 cups plain nonfat Greek yogurt, divided**
> **1 cup blueberries**
> **3 tablespoons sugar, divided**
> **6 (5-ounce) paper or plastic cups or pop molds**
> **1 cup sliced strawberries**
> **6 pop sticks**

1. Combine 1 cup yogurt, blueberries and 1½ tablespoons sugar in blender or food processor; blend until smooth.

2. Pour mixture into cups. Freeze 2 hours.

3. Combine strawberries, remaining 1 cup yogurt and 1½ tablespoons sugar in blender or food processor; blend until smooth.

4. Pour mixture into cups over blueberry layer. Cover top of each cup with small piece of foil. Freeze 2 hours.

5. Insert sticks through center of foil. Freeze 4 hours or until firm.

6. To serve, remove foil and peel away paper cups or gently twist frozen pops out of plastic cups.

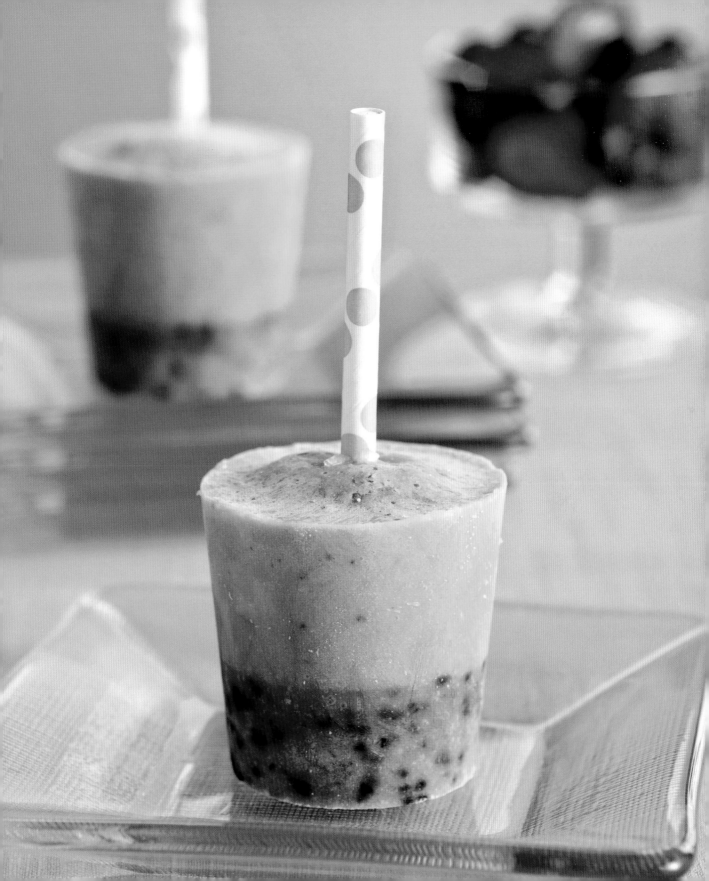

ASIAN PARTY MIX

Makes 10 cups (about 20 servings)

3 cups gluten-free rice cereal squares
3 cups gluten-free corn cereal squares
2 cups gluten-free mini pretzels
1 cup roasted salted soynuts
1 cup dry-roasted salted peanuts
5 tablespoons unsalted butter, melted
3 tablespoons gluten-free soy sauce
2 tablespoons packed brown sugar
2 tablespoons gluten-free teriyaki sauce
½ teaspoon ground ginger
½ teaspoon garlic salt
¼ teaspoon ground red pepper

1. Preheat oven to 250°F.

2. Combine cereals, pretzels, soynuts and peanuts in large bowl. Whisk butter, soy sauce, brown sugar, teriyaki sauce, ginger, garlic salt and ground red pepper in small bowl until smooth. Pour over cereal mixture; toss to coat evenly. Spoon mixture into 13×9-inch baking pan.

3. Bake 1 hour, stirring every 15 minutes. Spread on paper towels to cool completely. Store in airtight container.

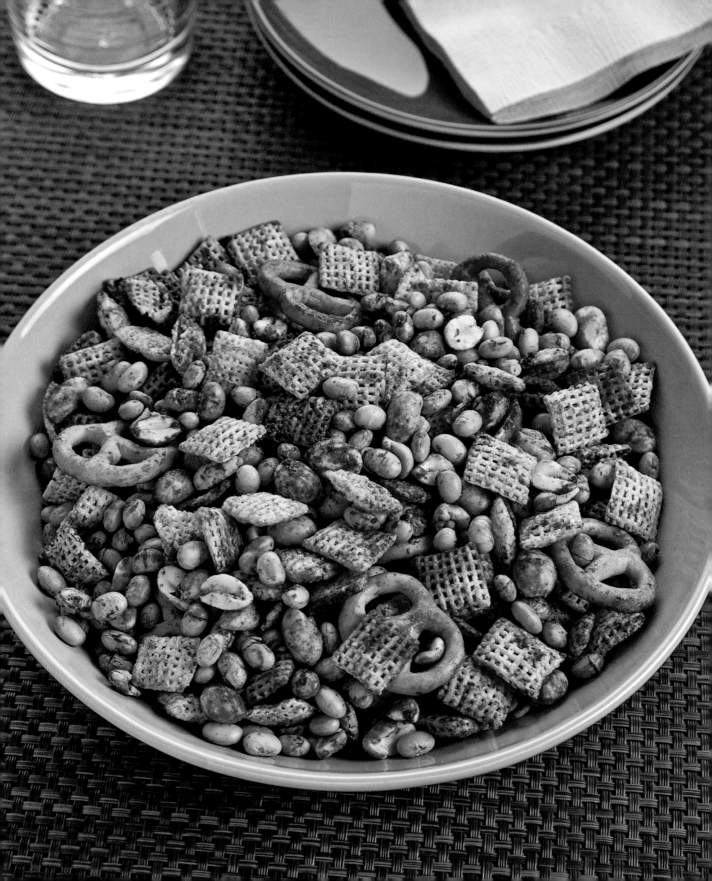

CITRUS CANDIED NUTS

Makes about 3 cups

>   1 egg white
> 1½ cups whole almonds
> 1½ cups pecan halves
>   1 cup powdered sugar
>   2 tablespoons lemon juice
>   2 teaspoons grated orange peel
>   1 teaspoon grated lemon peel
> ⅛ teaspoon ground nutmeg

1. Preheat oven to 300°F. Grease 15×10×1-inch jelly-roll pan.

2. Beat egg white in medium bowl with electric mixer at high speed until soft peaks form. Add almonds and pecans; stir until well coated. Stir in powdered sugar, lemon juice, orange peel, lemon peel and nutmeg until evenly coated. Spread nuts in single layer in prepared pan.

3. Bake 30 minutes, stirring after 20 minutes. Turn oven off. Let nuts stand in oven 15 minutes. Remove nuts from pan to sheet of foil. Cool completely. Store in airtight container up to 2 weeks.

ENERGY SMOOTHIE

Makes 4 servings

>   1 package (16 ounces) frozen unsweetened strawberries, partially thawed
>   2 ripe bananas, sliced
>   1 cup vanilla soymilk or milk*
>   1 container (6 ounces) vanilla nonfat Greek yogurt
> ⅓ cup powdered sugar
>   2 teaspoons vanilla

*If using milk, add 1 to 2 tablespoons additional sugar, if desired.

1. Combine strawberries, bananas, yogurt, soymilk, powdered sugar and vanilla in blender or food processor; blend until smooth.

2. Pour into four glasses. Serve immediately.

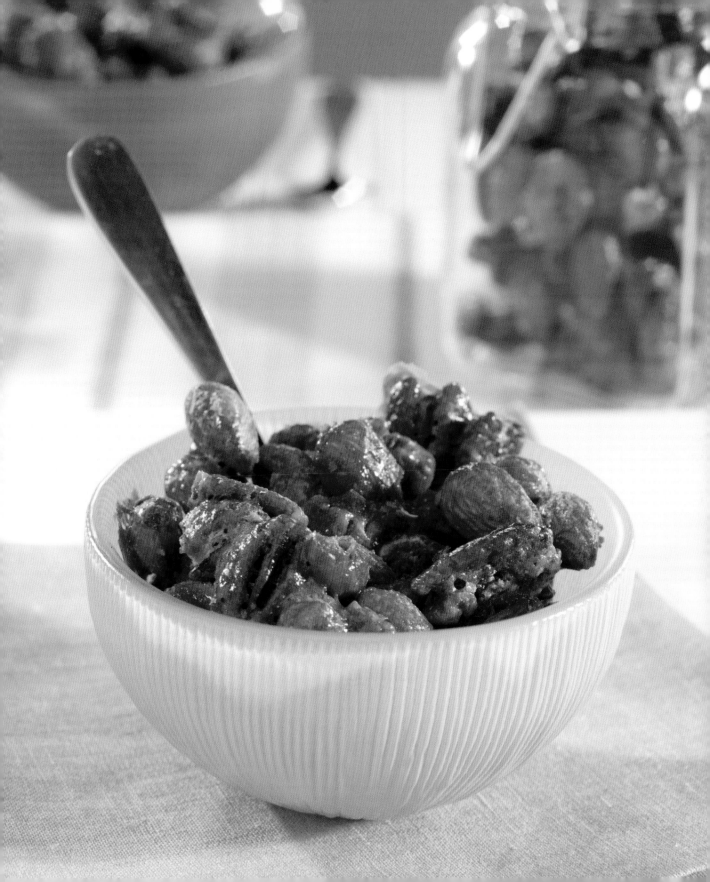

FRUIT KABOBS WITH RASPBERRY YOGURT DIP

Makes 6 servings

½ cup plain nonfat yogurt
¼ cup no-sugar-added raspberry fruit spread
1 pint fresh strawberries
2 cups cubed honeydew melon (1-inch cubes)
2 cups cubed cantaloupe (1-inch cubes)
1 can (8 ounces) pineapple chunks in juice, drained

1. Stir yogurt and fruit spread in small bowl until well blended.

2. Thread fruit alternately onto six 12-inch skewers. Serve with yogurt dip.

CINNAMON-HONEY POPS

Makes 6 pops

1¼ cups plain nonfat Greek yogurt
½ cup honey
¼ cup fat-free (skim) milk
1 tablespoon sugar
½ teaspoon ground cinnamon
½ teaspoon vanilla
Paper or plastic cups or pop molds
Pop sticks

1. Combine yogurt, honey, milk, sugar, cinnamon and vanilla in blender or food processor; blend until smooth.

2. Pour mixture into cups. Cover top of each cup with small piece of foil. Freeze 2 hours.*

3. Insert sticks through center of foil. Freeze 4 hours or until firm.

4. To serve, remove foil and peel away paper cups or gently twist frozen pops out of plastic cups.

*If using pop molds with lids, skip step 3 and freeze until firm.

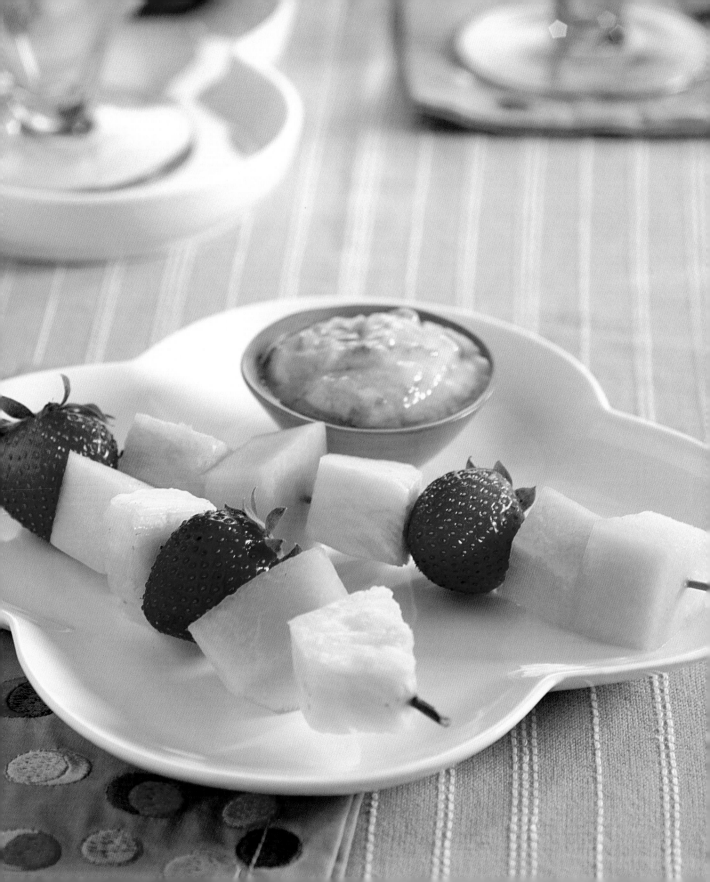

CHOCOLATE-ALMOND CRISPY TREATS

Makes 24 bars

> 6 cups gluten-free crisp brown rice cereal
> 1½ cups sliced almonds, toasted*
> 1 cup light corn syrup
> ⅓ cup almond butter
> ¼ cup packed brown sugar
> 3 tablespoons unsweetened cocoa powder
> ¼ teaspoon salt
> 1 cup semisweet chocolate chips

To toast almonds, spread in single layer in heavy skillet. Cook over medium heat 1 to 2 minutes or until nuts are lightly browned, stirring frequently.

1. Line 13×9-inch baking pan with parchment paper. Spray with nonstick cooking spray.

2. Combine rice cereal and almonds in large bowl; set aside.

3. Combine corn syrup, almond butter, brown sugar, cocoa and salt in large saucepan. Cook and stir over medium heat 5 minutes or until mixture is smooth and just begins to boil across surface. Remove from heat.

4. Immediately stir cereal mixture into saucepan. Gently fold in chocolate chips. Press firmly into prepared pan. Let stand 1 hour or until set. Cut into bars.

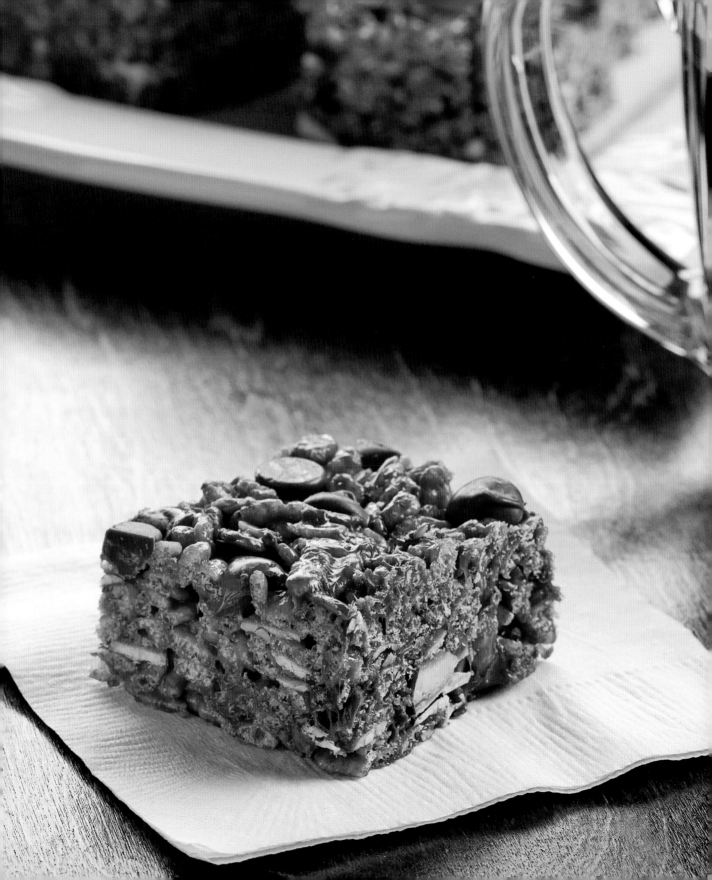

CHEDDAR CRACKERS

Makes 24 crackers (about 6 servings)

1½ cups brown rice flour
1 teaspoon garlic powder
1 teaspoon Italian seasoning
½ teaspoon salt
6 tablespoons (¾ stick) cold butter, cut into ½-inch cubes
½ cup (2 ounces) finely grated sharp Cheddar cheese
½ cup cold water

1. Combine brown rice flour, garlic powder, Italian seasoning and salt in food processor or blender; process until well blended. Add butter and cheese; pulse until coarse crumbs form. Add water; process until dough forms.

2. Divide dough into two pieces; wrap in plastic wrap and refrigerate 20 minutes.

3. Preheat oven to 350°F. Line baking sheets with parchment paper.

4. Place each dough half between two pieces of parchment paper; roll out to ¹⁄₁₆-inch thickness. Refrigerate 5 minutes.

5. Cut dough into 2½-inch squares; place on prepared baking sheets.

6. Bake 15 minutes or until golden and crisp, rotating baking sheets after 10 minutes. Cool on baking sheets 10 minutes. Remove to wire racks; cool completely.

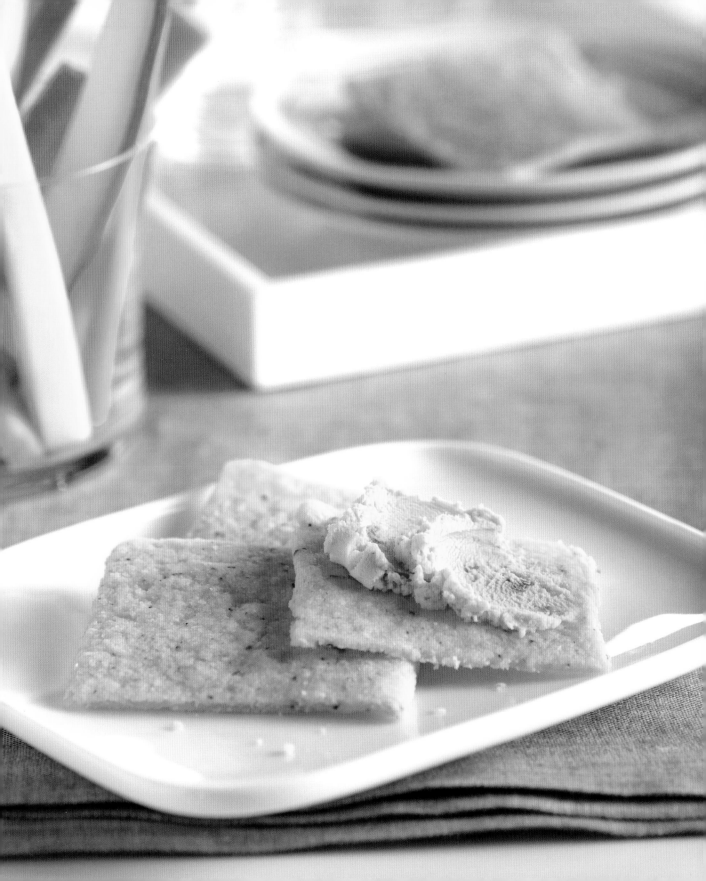

WASABI CREAM CHEESE SPREAD

Makes 1 cup (about 8 servings)

> 8 ounces low-fat cream cheese, softened
> 1 tablespoon wasabi paste
> 2 tablespoons fresh lime juice
> 2 teaspoons rice vinegar
> 2 tablespoons frozen shelled edamame, thawed
> 2 tablespoons chopped green onion, plus additional for garnish
> Rice crackers

1. Combine cream cheese, wasabi paste, lime juice and vinegar in small bowl; mix well. Fold in edamame and 2 tablespoons green onion.

2. Serve immediately or cover and refrigerate until ready to serve. Serve with rice crackers. Garnish with additional green onion.

CHEWY CORN BREAD COOKIES

Makes 4 dozen cookies

> 1 cup (2 sticks) unsalted butter, softened
> ⅔ cup plus 2 tablespoons sugar, divided
> 1 egg
> 1 teaspoon vanilla
> ½ teaspoon salt
> 2 cups corn flour
> ½ cup instant polenta

1. Beat butter and ⅔ cup sugar in large bowl with electric mixer at medium-high speed until creamy. Beat in egg, vanilla and salt until well blended. Combine corn flour and polenta in medium bowl. Gradually add to butter mixture, beating well after each addition. (Dough will be very sticky.)

2. Shape dough into two discs. Wrap in plastic wrap; refrigerate at least 2 hours.

3. Preheat oven to 350°F. Line cookie sheets with parchment paper. Shape dough into 1-inch balls. Roll in remaining 2 tablespoons sugar. Place 1 inch apart on prepared cookie sheets.

4. Bake 12 to 14 minutes. Cool completely on cookie sheets.

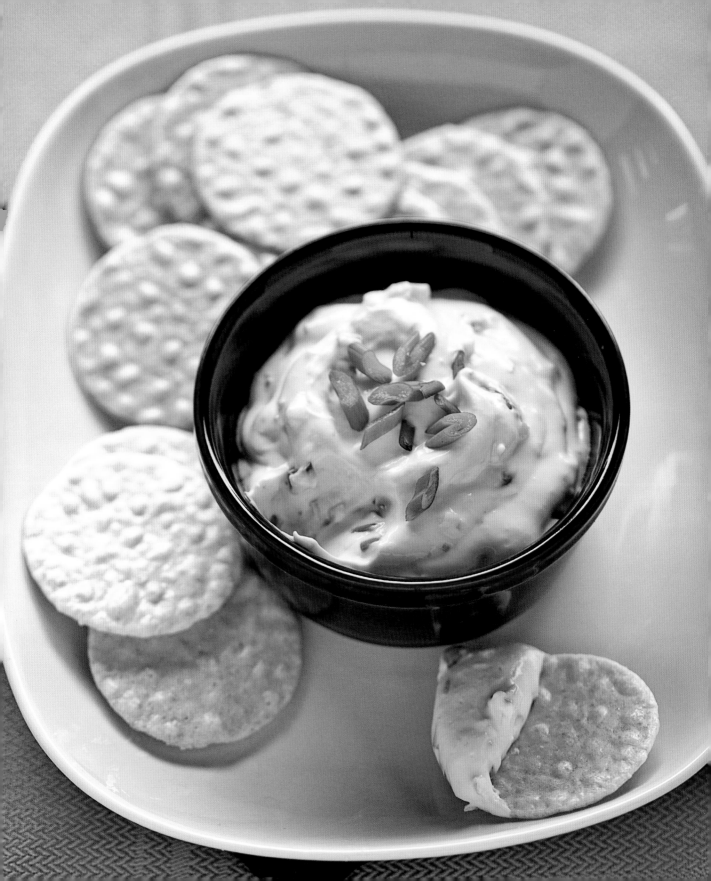

GRAHAM CRACKERS

Makes about 12 crackers (about 6 servings)

½ cup sweet rice flour (mochiko), plus additional for work surface
½ cup sorghum flour
½ cup packed brown sugar
⅓ cup tapioca flour
½ teaspoon baking soda
½ teaspoon salt
¼ cup (½ stick) butter or dairy-free margarine
2 tablespoons plus 2 teaspoons whole milk or dairy-free milk
2 tablespoons honey
1 tablespoon vanilla

1. Combine ½ cup sweet rice flour, sorghum flour, brown sugar, tapioca flour, baking soda and salt in food processor; pulse to combine, making sure brown sugar is free of lumps. Add butter; pulse until coarse crumbs form.

2. Whisk milk, honey and vanilla in small bowl or measuring cup until well blended and honey is dissolved. Pour into flour mixture; process until dough forms. (Dough will be very soft and sticky.)

3. Transfer dough to floured surface; pat into rectangle. Wrap in plastic wrap and refrigerate at least 4 hours or up to 2 days.

4. Preheat oven to 325°F. Cover work surface with parchment paper; generously dust with sweet rice flour.

5. Roll dough to ⅛-inch-thick rectangle on parchment paper using rice-floured rolling pin. (If dough becomes too sticky, return to refrigerator or freezer for several minutes.) Place dough on parchment paper on baking sheet. Score dough into cracker shapes (do not cut all the way through). Prick dough in rows with tines of fork. Place baking sheet in freezer 5 to 10 minutes or in refrigerator 15 to 20 minutes.

6. Bake chilled crackers 25 minutes or until firm and slightly darkened. Transfer parchment to wire rack to cool. Cut crackers when cooled slightly.

Serving Suggestion: Serve crackers as a snack or for s'mores with chocolate and marshmallows.

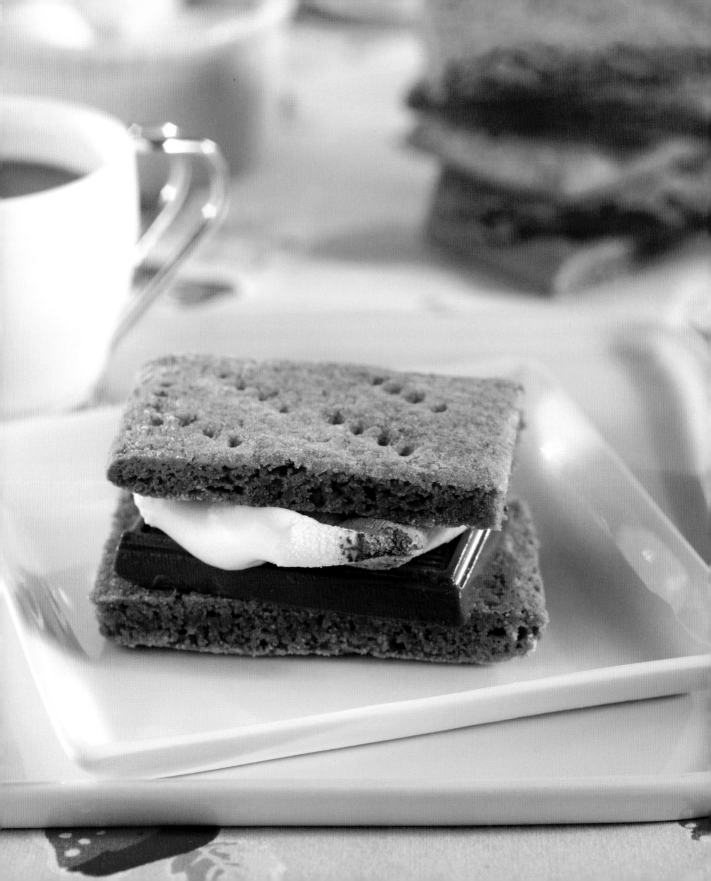

SWEET & SPICY POPCORN CLUSTERS

Makes 6 servings

½ cup sugar
6 tablespoons (¾ stick) butter
4 teaspoons light corn syrup
½ teaspoon salt
½ teaspoon ground red pepper
12 cups popped light butter-flavored microwave popcorn

1. Combine sugar, butter, corn syrup, salt and ground red pepper in large saucepan. Bring to a boil over medium heat; boil 3 minutes. Remove from heat.

2. Immediately stir in popcorn; toss to coat evenly.

3. Spread mixture in single layer on baking sheets. Let stand 1 hour to cool completely. Break into clusters. Store in airtight container.

TIP

One regular-size microwavable package of popcorn yields about 12 cups of popped popcorn.

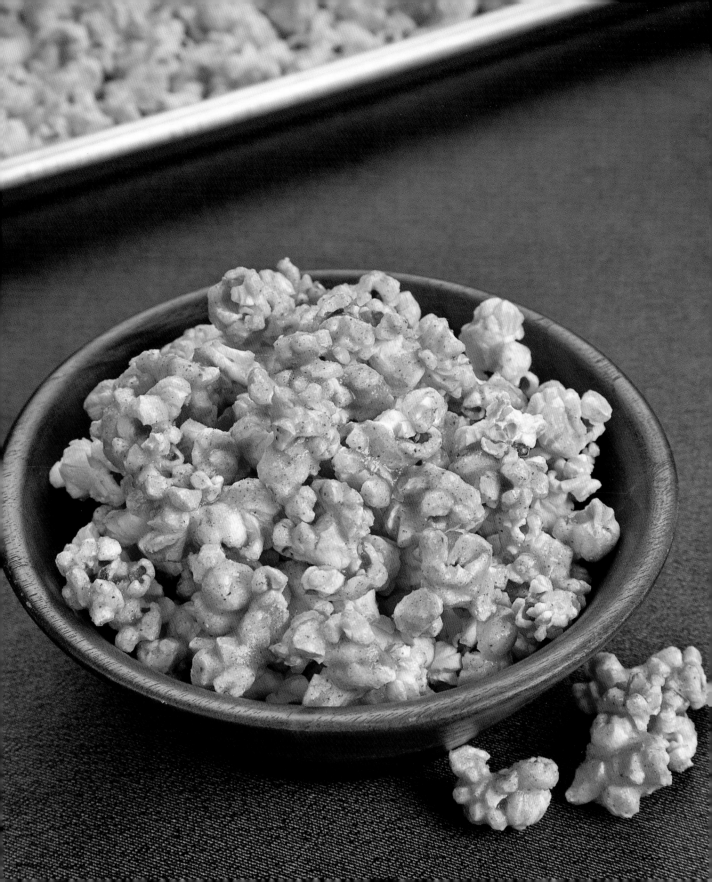

Kiddie Creations

HAM & OINKS

Makes 2 servings

>   2 teaspoons olive oil
>   2 eggs
>   Salt and black pepper
>   2 crisp corn tostada shells*
>   ¼ cup (1 ounce) shredded Mexican cheese blend (optional)
>   2 round deli ham slices, plus additional for decoration
>   Tomato slices
>   Squeezable yellow mustard

If prepared tostada shells are not available, crisp regular corn tortillas by brushing with oil and baking in a 350°F oven for 10 to 15 minutes.

1. Heat oil in small nonstick skillet over medium-low heat. Add eggs; season with salt and pepper. Scramble 2 to 3 minutes until firm.

2. Place tostada shells on serving plates. Divide egg mixture between tostada shells. Top eggs with shredded cheese, if desired. Arrange ham slices over eggs. Cut additional ham into triangle shapes for ears. Place oval tomato slice for nose. Use mustard to draw eyes and mouth.

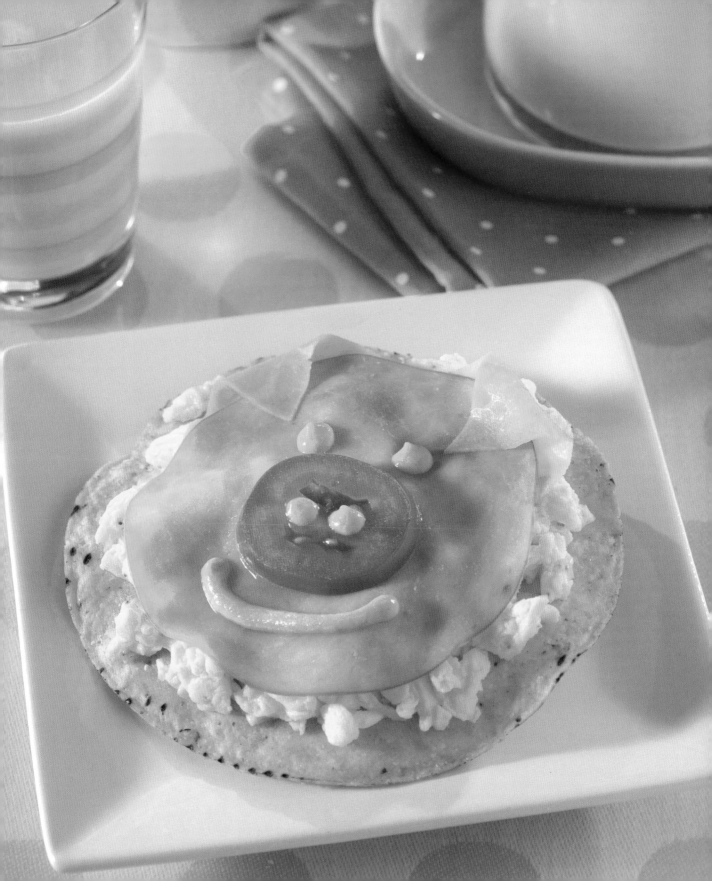

MEAT LOAF CUPCAKES

Makes 10 servings

  1½ pounds ground beef
   ½ cup finely chopped onion
   ⅓ cup crushed gluten-free corn or rice cereal squares
    1 egg
    2 tablespoons chopped fresh rosemary leaves
    3 medium potatoes, peeled and cut into 1-inch pieces
   ½ cup whole milk
    2 tablespoons butter
    1 teaspoon salt
     Black pepper
   ¼ cup snipped fresh chives

1. Preheat oven to 350°F.

2. Combine beef, onion, cereal, egg and rosemary in large bowl; mix well. Divide mixture evenly among 10 standard (2½-inch) muffin cups or silicone baking cups. Bake 25 minutes or until cooked through (160°F).

3. Meanwhile, place potatoes in medium saucepan; add enough water to cover. Bring to a boil; cook 20 to 25 minutes or until potatoes are very tender. Drain.

4. Beat potatoes, milk, butter, salt and pepper in large bowl with electric mixer at medium speed 3 minutes or until smooth. Place mashed potato mixture in large piping bag fitted with large star tip.

5. Remove meat loaf cupcakes to serving platter. Pipe mashed potatoes on top. Sprinkle with chives.

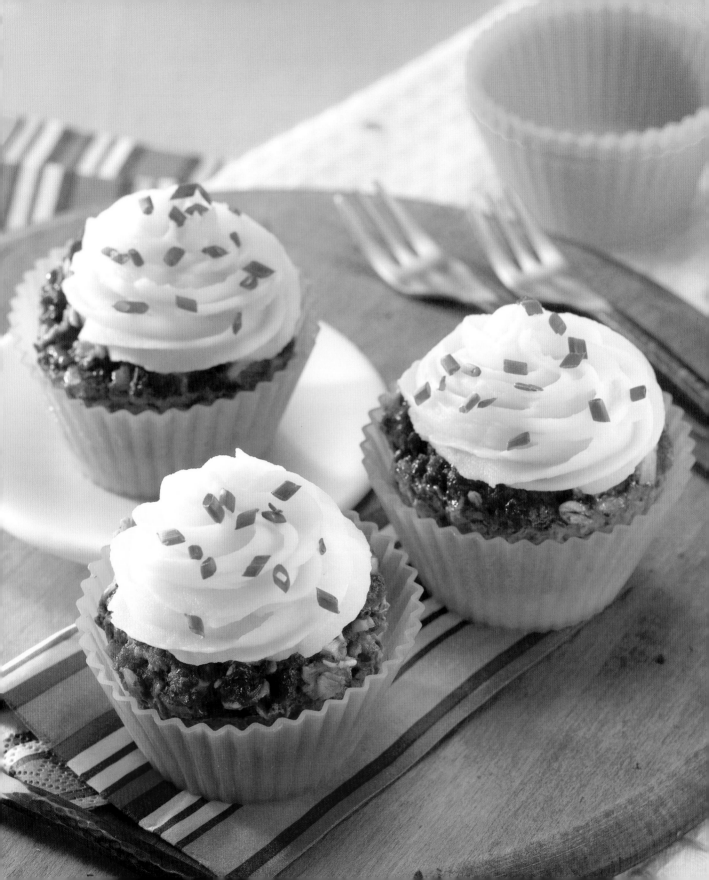

FARM-STYLE CASSEROLE

Makes 4 to 6 servings

   1 tablespoon canola oil
   1 small onion, chopped
   1 clove garlic, minced
   1 pound ground beef
   1 can (14½ ounces) diced tomatoes
   1 cup frozen corn
   1 cup frozen baby lima beans
   1 teaspoon salt
  ½ teaspoon dried oregano
  ¼ teaspoon black pepper
   2 cups cooked gluten-free macaroni or other pasta
   1 cup crushed corn tortilla chips

1. Preheat oven to 350°F. Heat oil in large nonstick skillet over medium heat. Add onion and garlic; cook and stir 5 to 6 minutes or until onion is tender. Add beef; brown 6 to 8 minutes, stirring to break up meat. Drain fat.

2. Stir in tomatoes, corn, lima beans, salt, oregano and pepper. Increase heat to high; cook and stir 5 minutes or until all liquid is evaporated. Stir in macaroni. Spoon mixture into 9-inch square baking dish. Sprinkle with tortilla chips.

3. Bake 20 minutes or until heated through.

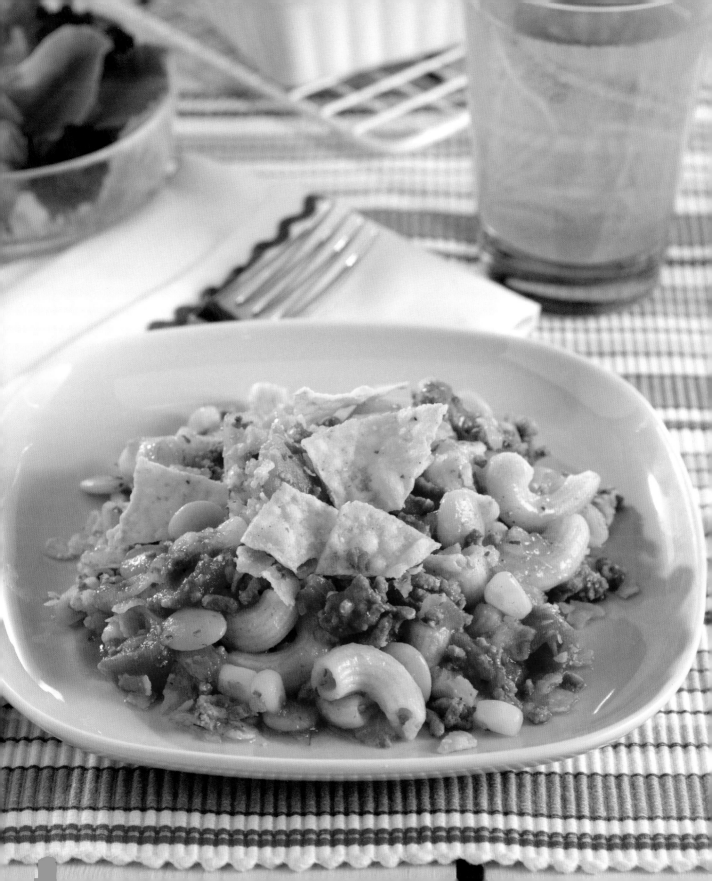

CARROT STIX

Makes 4 to 6 servings

    1 package (16 ounces) carrots
    2 teaspoons olive oil
    ½ teaspoon salt
    ¼ teaspoon black pepper
    1 teaspoon sugar
    ¼ teaspoon ground cinnamon

1. Preheat oven to 375°F. Line large baking sheet with foil.

2. Cut carrots in half crosswise. Cut each piece lengthwise into strips. Combine carrot sticks, oil, salt and pepper in large bowl. Toss to coat.

3. Arrange carrots on prepared baking sheet. Bake 20 minutes, turning once.

4. Meanwhile, combine sugar and cinnamon in small bowl.

5. Transfer baked carrots to large bowl. Sprinkle with sugar-cinnamon mixture; toss to coat. Serve immediately.

TIP

One bag (16 ounces) of baby carrots can be substituted for the large carrots. Bake for 25 minutes.

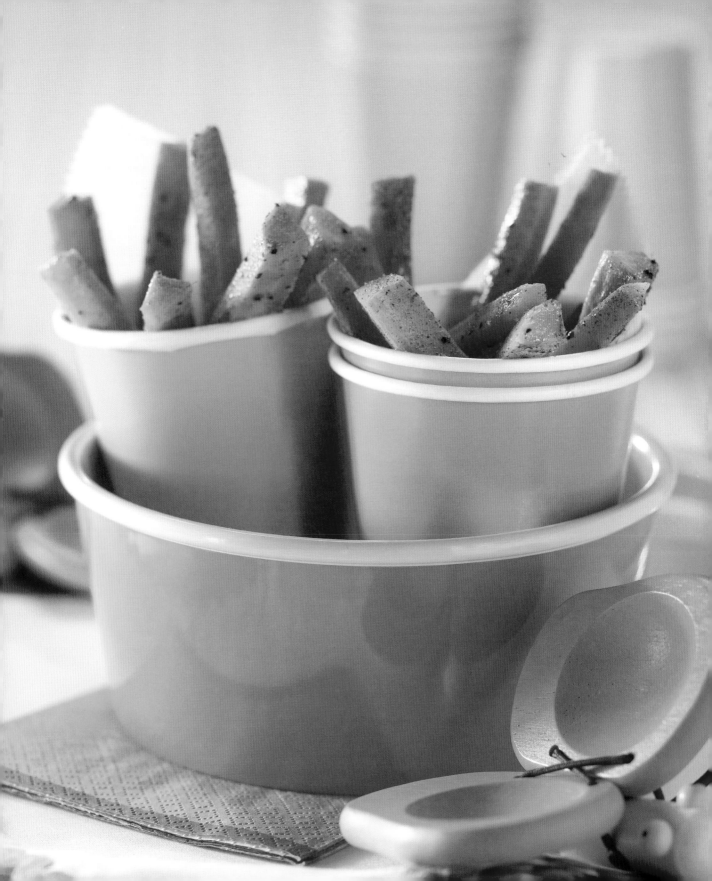

EXTRA CRUNCHY CHICKEN TENDERS

Makes 4 to 6 servings

  2 cups gluten-free corn flakes
  1 cup gluten-free pretzels
  ½ teaspoon garlic powder
  ⅛ teaspoon paprika
  ⅛ teaspoon dry mustard
  1 cup Gluten-Free All-Purpose Flour Blend (page 19)*
  1 teaspoon salt
  ½ teaspoon black pepper
  3 eggs, lightly beaten
  1 teaspoon gluten-free soy sauce
  1 pound chicken tenders
     Ketchup and/or honey mustard

*Or use any all-purpose gluten-free flour blend that does not contain xanthan gum.

1. Preheat oven to 350°F. Spray large baking sheet with nonstick cooking spray.

2. Combine corn flakes and pretzels in food processor; pulse until coarse crumbs form. Transfer crumbs to shallow dish; stir in garlic powder, paprika and mustard powder. Combine flour blend, salt and pepper in another shallow dish. Combine eggs and soy sauce in third shallow dish.

3. Dredge chicken tenders in flour mixture; shake off excess. Dip in egg mixture, letting excess drip back into dish. Coat in crumb mixture, pressing lightly to adhere.

4. Spray large nonstick skillet with cooking spray; heat over medium heat. Working in batches, brown chicken on both sides. Transfer to prepared baking sheet.

5. Bake 10 minutes or until golden brown. Serve with ketchup and/or honey mustard.

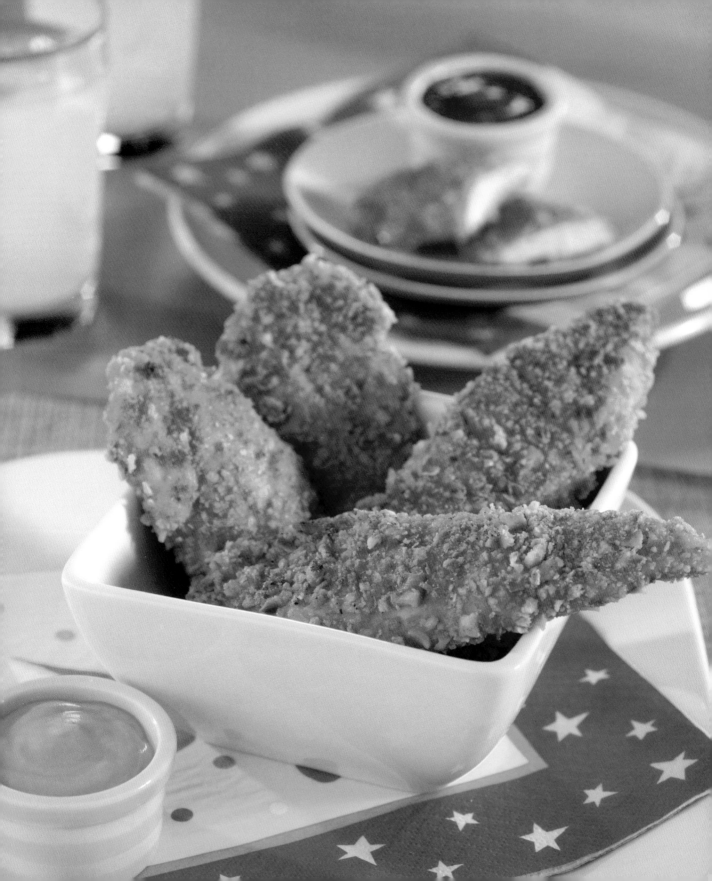

POLENTA STARS WITH BELL PEPPER SALSA

Makes 8 servings

    Bell Pepper Salsa (recipe follows)
4 cups water
1 tablespoon olive oil
1 teaspoon salt
1 cup yellow cornmeal
½ teaspoon chili powder
½ teaspoon garlic powder

1. Prepare Bell Pepper Salsa; set aside. Preheat oven to 375°F. Spray 13×9-inch baking pan with nonstick cooking spray.

2. Combine water, oil and salt in medium saucepan; bring to a boil. Combine cornmeal, chili powder and garlic powder in small bowl; slowly add to saucepan, stirring constantly to prevent clumps from forming. Reduce heat; simmer 20 minutes, stirring constantly. Spread polenta in prepared pan. Bake 25 minutes or until firm. Let stand 10 minutes.

3. Cut polenta into stars or other shapes with 2½-inch cookie cutters. Serve with Bell Pepper Salsa.

BELL PEPPER SALSA

Makes 2 cups

    1 cup chopped tomatoes
1 yellow or green bell pepper, chopped
2 jalapeño peppers,* seeded and finely chopped
2 tablespoons chopped fresh cilantro
2 tablespoons chopped onion
2 teaspoons red wine vinegar
¼ teaspoon salt

*Jalapeño peppers can sting and irritate the skin, so wear rubber gloves when handling peppers and do not touch your eyes.

Combine all ingredients in medium bowl.

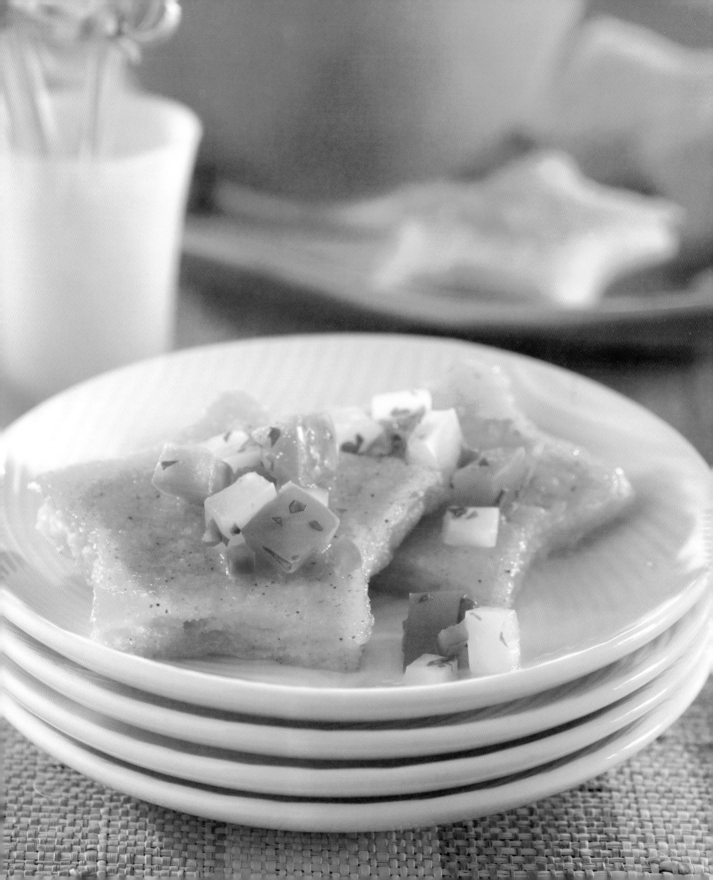

COWBOYS IN THE SADDLE

Makes 4 servings

    2 medium baking potatoes, cut into 8 wedges each
    ¾ teaspoon salt, divided
    ½ teaspoon black pepper, divided
    2 tablespoons canola oil
    1 pound skirt steak
    ¼ teaspoon dried oregano
       Gluten-free barbecue sauce, warmed

1. Preheat oven to 400°F. Place potato wedges on baking sheet. Sprinkle with ½ teaspoon salt and ¼ teaspoon pepper. Drizzle with oil. Bake 40 minutes or until golden brown and tender, turning once.

2. Season steak with remaining ¼ teaspoon salt, ¼ teaspoon pepper and oregano. Broil 4 inches from heat source 3 to 4 minutes per side or until desired doneness. Slice steak across the grain into 16 strips.

3. Arrange potato wedges on serving plates; drape slice of steak over each potato. Serve with barbecue sauce.

TIP

If desired, grill the skirt steak over medium-high heat 3 to 5 minutes per side.

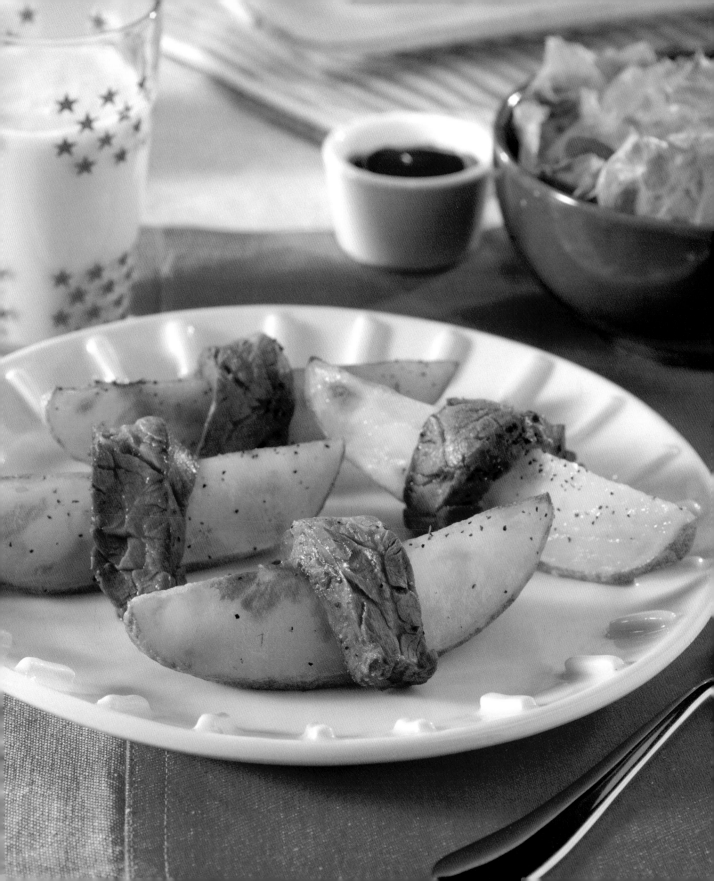

PB JOE & JANE

Makes 2 servings

> 2 rice cakes
> 2 tablespoons smooth peanut butter
> 1 red apple
>   Apricot, grape or cherry preserves
>   Grapes
>   Dried cranberries

Place rice cakes on work surface. Spread with peanut butter. Cut apple into short sticks for Joe's hair. Cut apple triangles for mouths. Make Jane's hair with preserves. Slice grape into halves for Joe's eyes. Add cranberries for Jane's hair and eyes and Joe's nose.

HIP HOP HASH

Makes 4 servings

> 1 tablespoon butter
> 1 tablespoon sweet rice flour (mochiko)
> ⅓ cup gluten-free beef broth
> 1 teaspoon gluten-free Worcestershire sauce
> 1 pound beef pot roast, cooked and diced
> 1 medium sweet potato (about 12 ounces), peeled and diced
> 1 stalk celery, diced
> 1 cup corn
> ¼ cup diced red or green bell pepper
> ¼ cup (1 ounce) shredded Cheddar cheese (optional)

1. Melt butter in large skillet over medium heat. Whisk in sweet rice flour; cook 2 minutes, stirring constantly. Whisk in broth and Worcestershire sauce; bring to a simmer. Add beef, sweet potato, celery, corn and bell pepper. Return to a simmer; cover and cook 12 minutes or until vegetables are tender.

2. Sprinkle cheese over hash just before serving, if desired.

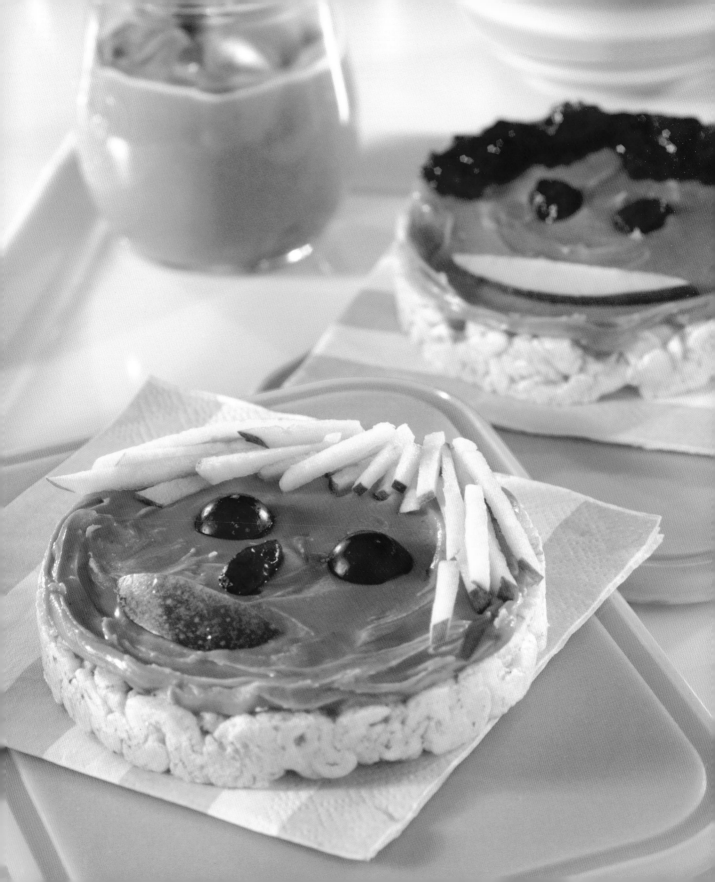

CHILI-TOPPED POTATO BOATS

Makes 6 servings

- 1 tablespoon canola oil
- 1 small onion, chopped
- 1 small green bell pepper, chopped
- 1 clove garlic, minced
- 1 pound ground beef
- 1 can (about 15 ounces) pinto or kidney beans, rinsed and drained
- 1 cup crushed tomatoes
- 1 tablespoon tomato paste
- ½ teaspoon ground cumin
- 1 teaspoon chili powder
- ¼ teaspoon chipotle chili powder
- ¾ teaspoon salt
- ¼ teaspoon black pepper
- 3 large baking potatoes, baked, halved lengthwise and scooped out

1. Heat oil in large nonstick skillet over medium heat. Add onion, bell pepper and garlic; cook and stir 5 to 6 minutes or until onion is tender. Add beef; brown 6 to 8 minutes, stirring to break up meat. Drain fat.

2. Stir in beans, tomatoes, tomato paste, cumin, chili powder, chipotle chili powder, salt and black pepper. Simmer 10 to 15 minutes or until chili is heated through and thickened. Spoon about ⅔ cup mixture into each potato half.

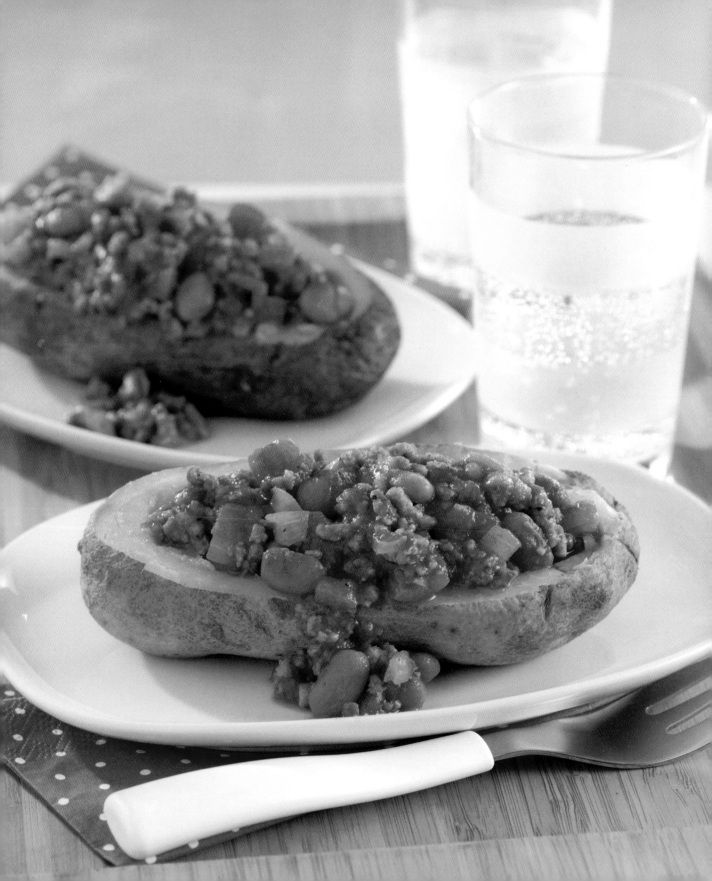

CORNY CRITTERS

Makes 10 to 12 pancakes (about 4 servings)

 1 cup yellow cornmeal
 1 tablespoon sugar
 ½ teaspoon salt
 1 cup boiling water
   Dried apricots
   Sliced almonds
 ½ cup Gluten-Free All-Purpose Flour Blend (page 19)*
 ½ cup soymilk or other dairy-free milk
 1 egg, beaten
 2 tablespoons dairy-free margarine, melted
 2 teaspoons baking powder
   Vegetable oil
   Dried cranberries
   Maple syrup (optional)

Or use any gluten-free all-purpose flour blend that does not contain xanthan gum.

1. Combine cornmeal, sugar and salt in medium bowl. Stir in boiling water. Cover; let stand 10 minutes. Cut apricots into shapes for noses, mouths and whiskers.

2. Stir flour blend, soymilk, egg, margarine and baking powder into cornmeal mixture until smooth. Transfer some of batter to measuring cup with pour spout.

3. Heat large nonstick skillet or griddle over medium heat. Brush lightly with oil.

4. Pour small circles of batter onto skillet; drizzle additional batter to make puppy or bunny ears. Use a knife to straighten edges of batter as needed. Add almonds and dried cranberries for eyes. Place triangular pieces of dried apricot for noses and curved lines for mouths. Press into batter.

5. Cook 2 to 3 minutes or until bubbles appear on top of pancakes and edges become dull. Turn carefully with spatula sprayed with nonstick cooking spray. Cook 1 to 2 minutes until lightly browned on both sides. Serve pancakes with maple syrup, if desired.

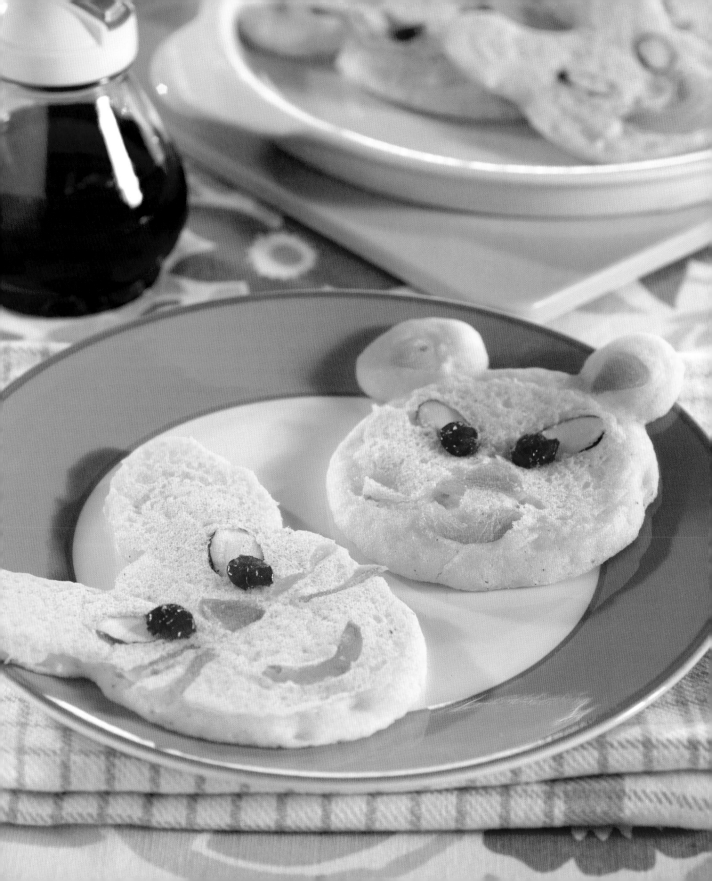

Allergy-Free Fare

POWER-PACKED SNACK BARS

Makes 16 bars

   3 cups puffed millet cereal
   1 cup chopped dried fruit
   ¼ cup roasted unsalted sunflower kernels
   1 teaspoon ground cinnamon
   ½ cup creamy soynut butter
   ½ cup honey
   2 tablespoons packed brown sugar

1. Line 8- to 9-inch square baking pan with parchment paper. Spray with nonstick cooking spray.

2. Combine cereal, dried fruit, sunflower kernels and cinnamon in large bowl; mix well.

3. Combine soynut butter, honey and brown sugar in small microwavable bowl. Microwave on HIGH 15 seconds or until melted and smooth.

4. Stir soynut butter mixture into millet mixture until well combined and evenly coated. Press firmly into prepared pan. Cover and refrigerate at least 2 hours or until firm. Cut into bars.

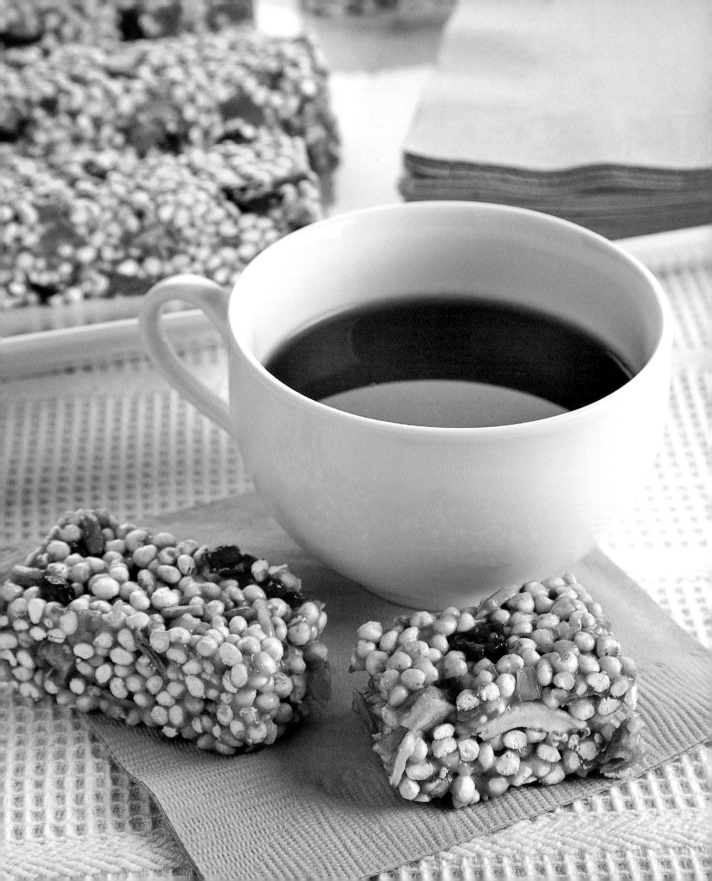

TUNA NOODLE BAKE

Makes 6 to 8 servings

4 tablespoons dairy-free margarine, divided
1 small onion, finely chopped
2 cloves garlic, minced
2 tablespoons sweet rice flour (mochiko)
1½ cups soymilk or other dairy-free milk
1 teaspoon Italian seasoning
½ teaspoon salt
½ teaspoon pepper
½ teaspoon dry mustard
½ teaspoon dried thyme
4 cups cooked gluten-free macaroni, rotini or other small pasta
2 cans (5 ounces each) tuna, drained and flaked
2 cups peas
½ cup crushed potato chips

1. Preheat oven to 350°F. Melt 2 tablespoons margarine in small skillet. Add onion and garlic; cook and stir 2 minutes or until softened.

2. Melt remaining 2 tablespoons margarine in medium saucepan over low heat. Whisk in sweet rice flour; cook 2 minutes, stirring constantly. Stir in soymilk; bring to a boil. Reduce heat; simmer 2 to 3 minutes or until thickened. Stir in Italian seasoning, salt, pepper, mustard and thyme.

3. Combine pasta, onion mixture, tuna and peas in large bowl. Stir in sauce until combined. Transfer to shallow baking dish or casserole. Sprinkle with potato chips.

4. Bake, covered, 15 minutes. Uncover; bake 10 minutes or until hot and bubbly.

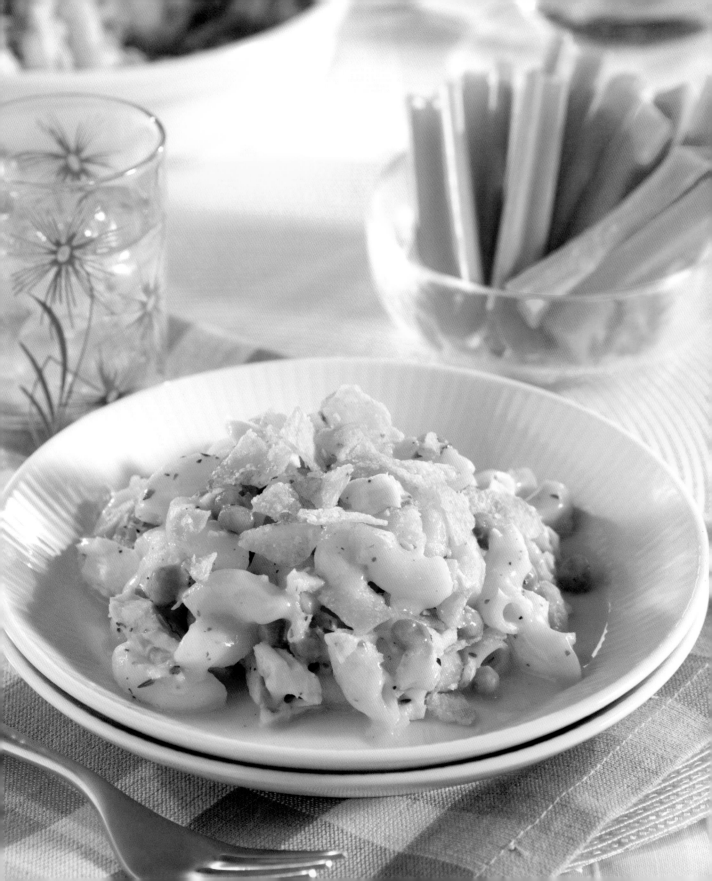

ALLERGY-FREE STRAWBERRY CAKE

Makes 8 servings

> 1 package (15 ounces) gluten-free yellow cake mix
> ½ cup rice milk
> ½ cup dairy-free margarine
> Prepared powdered egg replacer equal to 3 eggs
> 2 teaspoons grated lemon peel
> 1 teaspoon vanilla
> 1 cup sliced strawberries, plus additional for garnish
> 1 to 2 tablespoons powdered sugar

1. Preheat oven to 350°F. Spray 9-inch round cake pan with nonstick cooking spray.

2. Beat cake mix, rice milk, margarine, egg replacer, lemon peel and vanilla in large bowl with electric mixer at low speed 30 seconds. Increase speed to medium and beat 1 minute. Add 1 cup strawberries; beat at medium speed 1 to 2 minutes or until strawberries are crushed. Pour batter into prepared pan.

3. Bake 35 to 40 minutes or until golden brown and firm to the touch. Cool in pan 10 minutes. Remove wire rack to cool completely. Dust with powdered sugar. Garnish with additional strawberries.

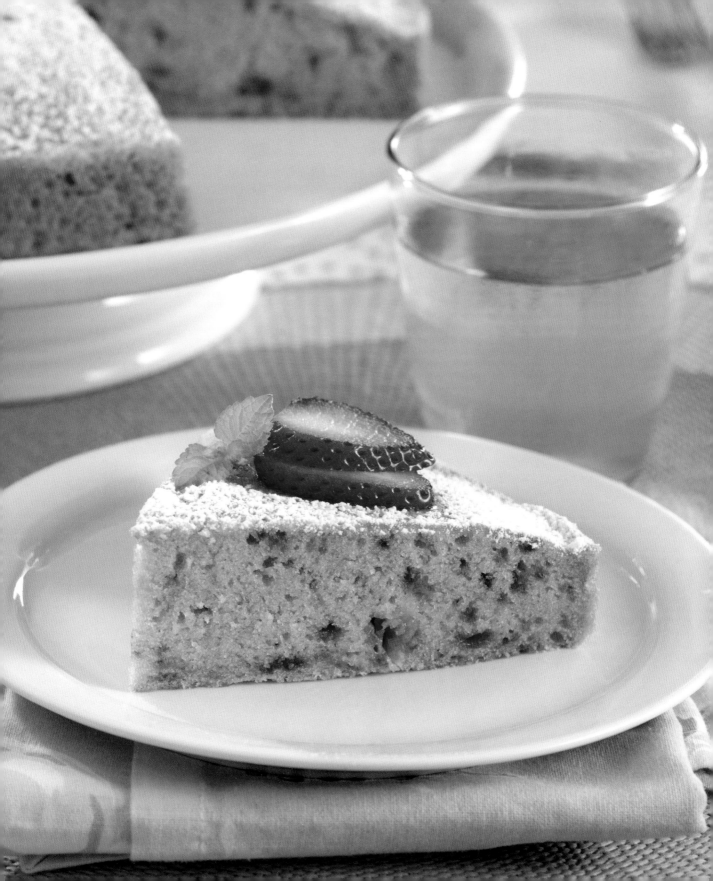

ALMOND BUTTER

Makes 2 cups (about 16 servings)

   1 package (16 ounces) roasted unsalted almonds
¼ cup canola oil, plus additional if desired
¼ cup honey, plus additional if desired
½ teaspoon salt

1. Grate almonds twice in food processor using grater disk. Remove almonds to large bowl. Remove grater disk; fit with metal blade.

2. Return almonds to food processor; process 2 to 3 minutes or until nuts clump together and form thick paste, scraping side of bowl occasionally.

3. With motor running, add oil, honey and salt through feed tube; process until desired consistency is reached, adding additional oil and honey, if desired. Store in airtight container.

INTENSE CHOCOLATE ICE CREAM

Makes 4 servings

   2 cups rice milk
¼ cup tapioca flour
¼ cup unsweetened cocoa powder
  6 tablespoons granulated sugar
¼ teaspoon salt
⅓ cup dairy-free chocolate chips
½ teaspoon vanilla

1. Whisk ½ cup rice milk, tapioca flour and cocoa in medium saucepan until smooth. Whisk in remaining 1½ cups rice milk, sugar and salt. Cook over medium heat until mixture thickens to consistency of pudding, stirring constantly.

2. Remove from heat. Add chocolate chips and vanilla; stir until chips are melted and mixture is smooth.

3. Transfer to medium bowl; cover and refrigerate 2 hours or until chilled.

4. Pour chocolate mixture into ice cream maker; process according to manufacturer's directions.

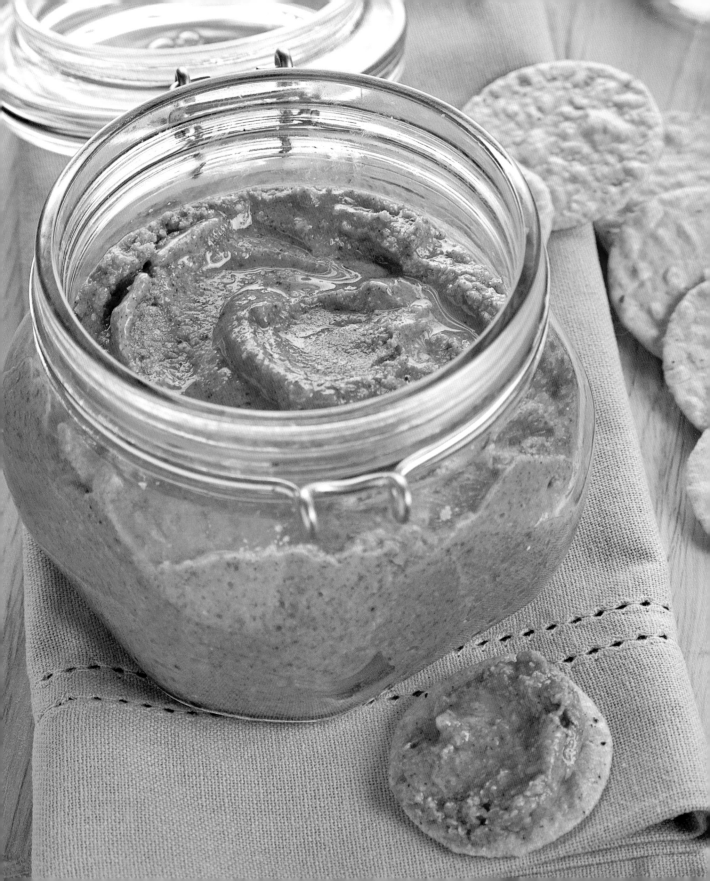

BLUEBERRY PANCAKE SMILES

Makes about 16 small pancakes (about 4 servings)

½ cup sorghum flour
¼ cup brown rice flour
¼ cup buckwheat flour
2 tablespoons sugar
2 teaspoons baking powder
⅛ teaspoon xanthan gum
1 to 1¼ cups rice milk
 Prepared powdered egg replacer equal to 1 egg
2 tablespoons vegetable oil
1 cup blueberries
 Maple syrup

1. Combine sorghum flour, brown rice flour, buckwheat flour, sugar, baking powder and xanthan gum in medium bowl. Whisk in rice milk, egg replacer and oil until dry ingredients are moistened.

2. Spray large skillet with nonstick cooking spray; heat over medium heat. Spoon batter into skillet 1 tablespoon at a time. Arrange blueberries on batter as desired. Cook 1 to 2 minutes or until lightly browned and edges begin to bubble. Turn over; cook 1 minute or until lightly browned. Serve with maple syrup, if desired.

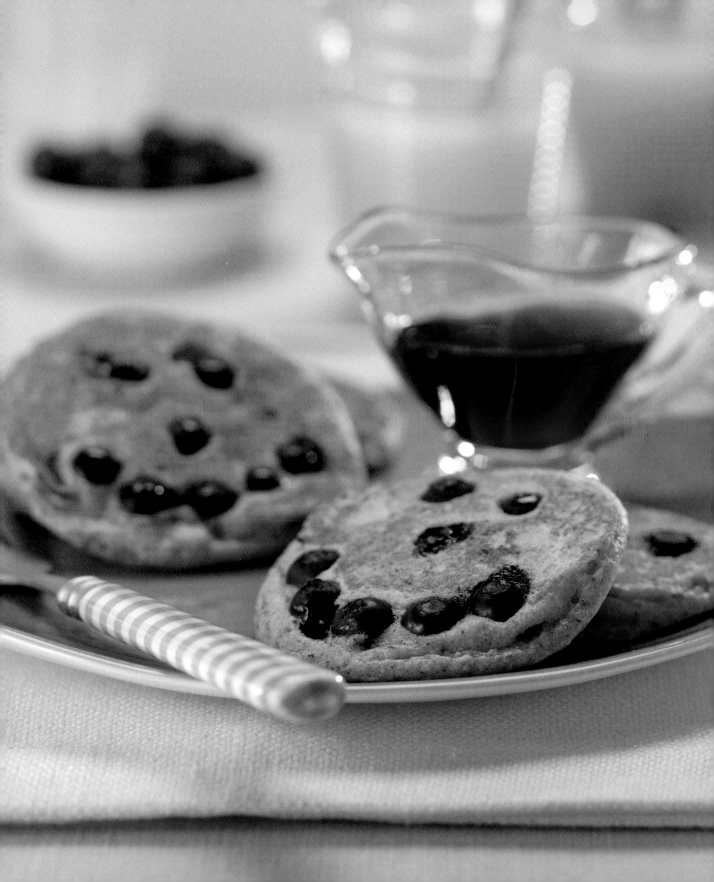

OVEN-FRIED CHICKEN

Makes 4 to 6 servings

   6 boneless skinless chicken thighs (about 1 pound)
½ cup rice milk
½ cup corn flour
1½ cups crushed gluten-free cornflakes
½ teaspoon salt
¼ teaspoon garlic powder
½ teaspoon paprika
¼ teaspoon black pepper
2 tablespoons dairy-free soy-free spread, melted

1. Place chicken in medium bowl. Add rice milk; cover and refrigerate 1 hour.

2. Preheat oven to 350°F. Spray rimmed baking sheet with nonstick cooking spray. Place corn flour in shallow dish. Combine cornflakes, salt, garlic powder, paprika and pepper in separate shallow dish.

3. Drain chicken; discard rice milk. Pat chicken dry. Lightly dust chicken with corn flour. Brush with melted spread. Coat chicken in cornflake mixture, pressing lightly to adhere. Arrange on prepared baking sheet.

4. Bake 35 to 40 minutes or until cooked through, turning halfway through.

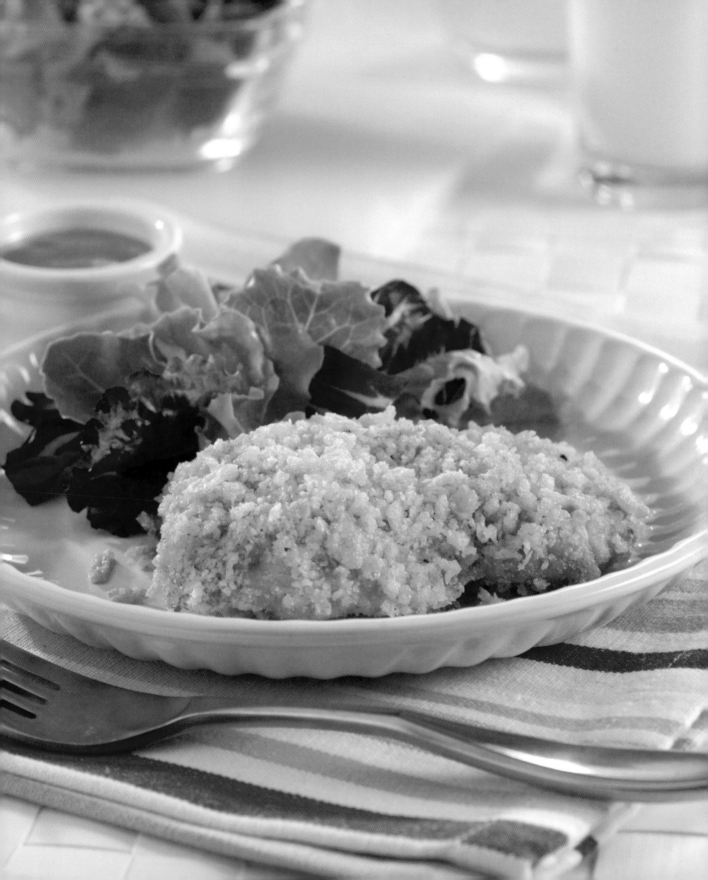

ALLERGY-FREE MAC & CHEEZ

Makes 4 servings

    8 ounces gluten-free elbows, rotini or other small pasta
    2 tablespoons flaked nutritional yeast*
    4 teaspoons sweet rice flour (mochiko)
    ½ teaspoon onion powder
    ½ teaspoon garlic powder
    ¾ teaspoon salt
    ¼ teaspoon dry mustard
    ½ cup soymilk or other dairy-free milk
    1 cup chopped cooked chicken (optional)
    1 cup cooked peas and/or chopped carrots (optional)

*Nutritional yeast can be found in health food stores and some supermarkets. It is NOT similar to regular yeast or brewer's yeast.

1. Bring large saucepan of water to a boil. Add pasta; cook 6 minutes or until al dente. Reserve ½ cup pasta cooking water; drain pasta. Oil pasta lightly if necessary to prevent sticking.

2. Meanwhile, combine nutritional yeast, sweet rice flour, onion powder, garlic powder, salt and mustard in small bowl; mix well.

3. Whisk nutritional yeast mixture into soymilk in large saucepan until smooth. Add pasta; cook and stir over medium heat 1 to 2 minutes. Add 4 to 6 tablespoons pasta cooking water and continue cooking 2 minutes or until sauce coats pasta and desired consistency is reached. Add chicken and/or vegetables, if desired; cook until heated through.

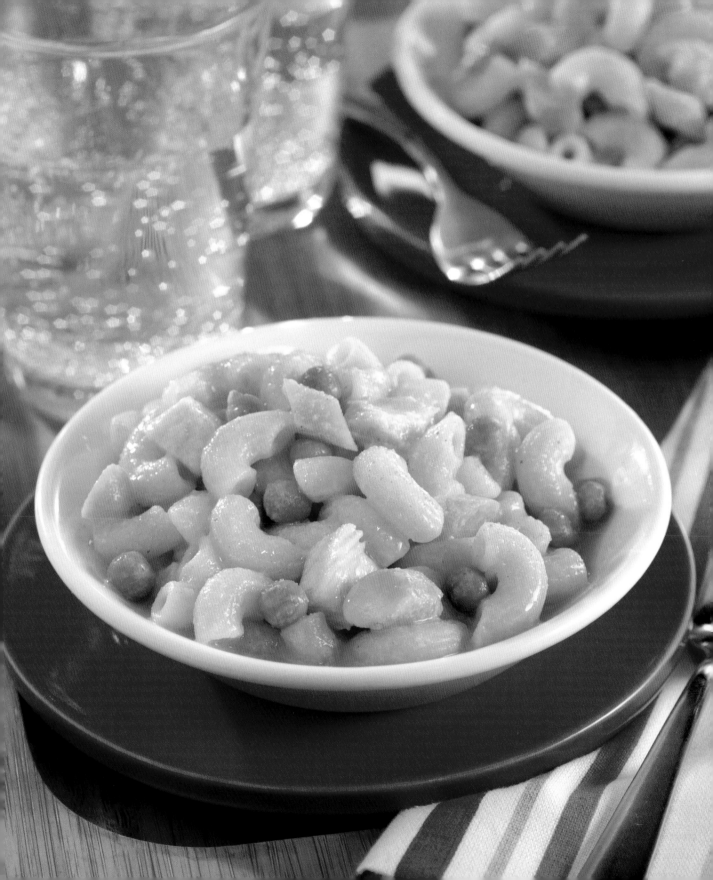

OLD-FASHIONED CHOCOLATE CHIP COOKIES

Makes about 4 dozen cookies

    3 tablespoons water
    1 tablespoon ground flax seed*
1⅓ cups Gluten-Free All-Purpose Flour Blend (page 19)**
    ½ teaspoon xanthan gum
    ½ teaspoon baking soda
    ½ teaspoon salt
    1 cup (2 sticks) dairy-free margarine, softened
    ½ cup granulated sugar
    ¼ cup packed brown sugar
1½ teaspoons vanilla
    1 cup dairy-free chocolate chips
    ½ cup roasted unsalted sunflower kernels

*This recipe can easily be made by substituting 1 egg for the ground flax seed and water.
**Or use any all-purpose gluten-free flour blend that does not contain xanthan gum.

1. Bring water and flax seed to a boil in small saucepan over medium-low heat. Simmer 5 minutes or until thickened. Cool completely.

2. Preheat oven to 350°F. Line baking sheets with parchment paper.

3. Combine flour blend, xanthan gum, baking soda and salt in medium bowl. Beat margarine, granulated sugar and brown sugar in large bowl with electric mixer at medium speed until smooth. Add flax seed mixture and vanilla; beat until well blended. Beat in flour mixture until combined. Fold in chocolate chips and sunflower kernels.

4. Drop dough by rounded tablespoonfuls 2 inches apart on prepared baking sheets.

5. Bake 10 to 12 minutes or until cookies are lightly browned. Cool on baking sheet 5 minutes. Remove to wire racks; cool completely.

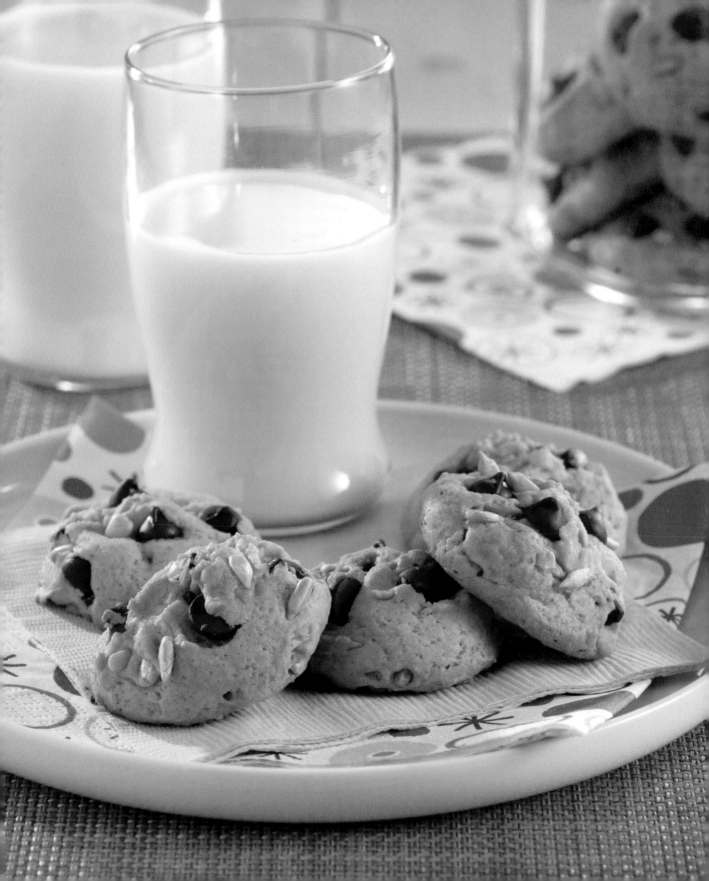

SCRAMBLED TOFU AND POTATOES

Makes 4 servings

Potatoes

 ¼ cup olive oil
 4 to 5 red potatoes, cubed
 ½ white onion, sliced
 1 tablespoon chopped fresh rosemary
 1 teaspoon coarse salt

Scrambled Tofu

 ¼ cup nutritional yeast*
 ½ teaspoon turmeric
 2 tablespoons water
 2 tablespoons gluten-free soy sauce
 1 package (14 ounces) firm tofu
 2 teaspoons olive oil
 ½ cup chopped green bell pepper
 ½ cup chopped red onion

*Nutritional yeast can be found in health food stores and some supermarkets. It is NOT similar to regular yeast or brewer's yeast.

1. For potatoes, preheat oven to 450°F. Place ¼ cup olive oil in 12-inch cast-iron skillet; place skillet in oven 10 minutes to heat.

2. Bring large saucepan of water to a boil. Add potatoes; cook 5 to 7 minutes or until fork-tender. Drain potatoes; return to saucepan. Stir in white onion, rosemary and salt. Spread mixture in preheated skillet. Bake 25 to 30 minutes or until potatoes are browned, stirring every 10 minutes.

3. For tofu, combine nutritional yeast and turmeric in small bowl. Stir in water and soy sauce until smooth.

4. Cut tofu into eight cubes. Gently squeeze out water; loosely crumble tofu into medium bowl. Heat 2 teaspoons olive oil in large skillet over medium-high heat. Add bell pepper and red onion; cook and stir 2 minutes or until soft but not browned. Add tofu; drizzle with 3 tablespoons nutritional yeast sauce. Cook and stir about 5 minutes or until liquid is evaporated and tofu is heated through. Stir in additional sauce, if desired, for stronger flavor.

5. Divide potatoes among four serving plates. Top with tofu mixture.

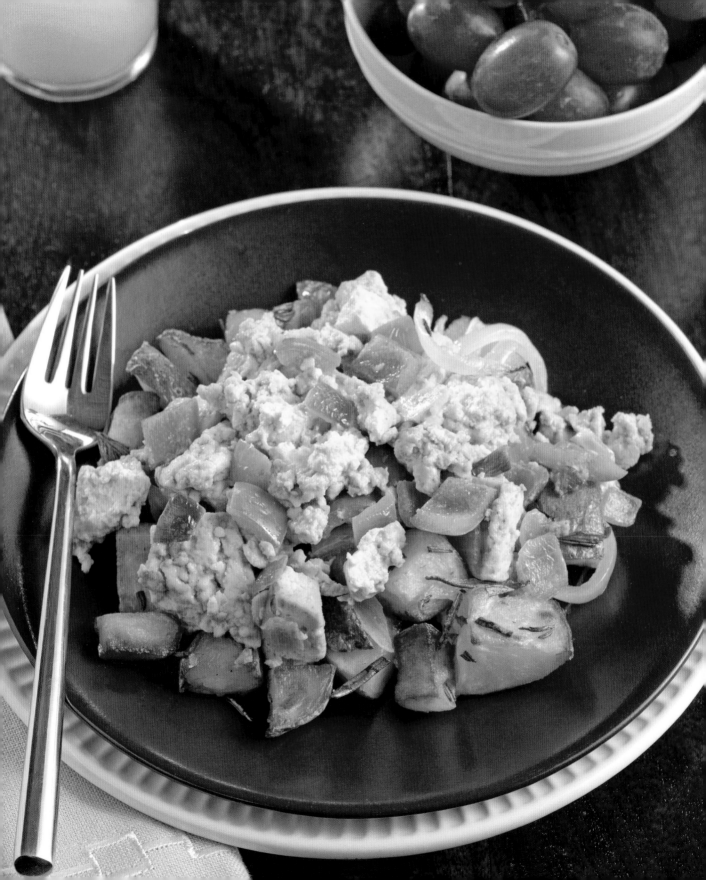

CRISP OATS TRAIL MIX

Makes 2½ cups (about 10 servings)

  1 cup gluten-free old-fashioned oats
  ½ cup unsalted shelled pumpkin seeds
  ½ cup dried sweetened cranberries
  ½ cup raisins
  2 tablespoons maple syrup
  1 teaspoon canola oil
  ½ teaspoon ground cinnamon
  ¼ teaspoon salt

1. Preheat oven to 325°F. Line baking sheet with heavy-duty foil.

2. Combine all ingredients in large bowl; mix well. Spread on prepared baking sheet.

3. Bake 20 minutes or until oats are lightly browned, stirring halfway through. Cool completely on baking sheet. Store in airtight container.

TIP

Shelled pumpkin seeds are also know as pepitas. They are often sold in the Mexican food section of the grocery store.

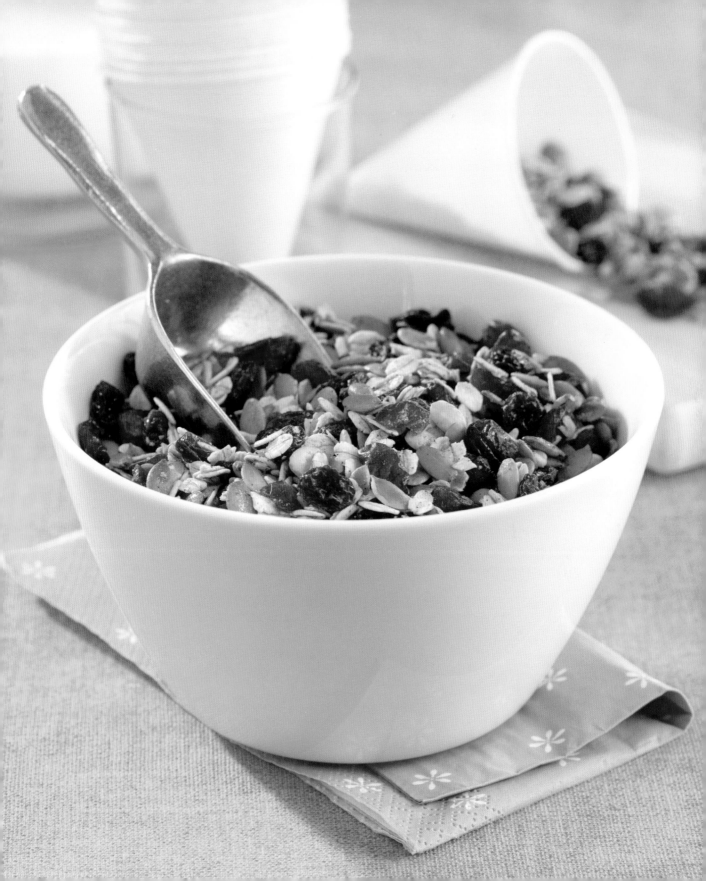

METRIC CONVERSION CHART

VOLUME MEASUREMENTS (dry)

1/8 teaspoon = 0.5 mL
1/4 teaspoon = 1 mL
1/2 teaspoon = 2 mL
3/4 teaspoon = 4 mL
1 teaspoon = 5 mL
1 tablespoon = 15 mL
2 tablespoons = 30 mL
1/4 cup = 60 mL
1/3 cup = 75 mL
1/2 cup = 125 mL
2/3 cup = 150 mL
3/4 cup = 175 mL
1 cup = 250 mL
2 cups = 1 pint = 500 mL
3 cups = 750 mL
4 cups = 1 quart = 1 L

VOLUME MEASUREMENTS (fluid)

1 fluid ounce (2 tablespoons) = 30 mL
4 fluid ounces (1/2 cup) = 125 mL
8 fluid ounces (1 cup) = 250 mL
12 fluid ounces (1 1/2 cups) = 375 mL
16 fluid ounces (2 cups) = 500 mL

WEIGHTS (mass)

1/2 ounce = 15 g
1 ounce = 30 g
3 ounces = 90 g
4 ounces = 120 g
8 ounces = 225 g
10 ounces = 285 g
12 ounces = 360 g
16 ounces = 1 pound = 450 g

DIMENSIONS

1/16 inch = 2 mm
1/8 inch = 3 mm
1/4 inch = 6 mm
1/2 inch = 1.5 cm
3/4 inch = 2 cm
1 inch = 2.5 cm

OVEN TEMPERATURES

250°F = 120°C
275°F = 140°C
300°F = 150°C
325°F = 160°C
350°F = 180°C
375°F = 190°C
400°F = 200°C
425°F = 220°C
450°F = 230°C

BAKING PAN SIZES

Utensil	Size in Inches/Quarts	Metric Volume	Size in Centimeters
Baking or Cake Pan (square or rectangular)	8×8×2	2 L	20×20×5
	9×9×2	2.5 L	23×23×5
	12×8×2	3 L	30×20×5
	13×9×2	3.5 L	33×23×5
Loaf Pan	8×4×3	1.5 L	20×10×7
	9×5×3	2 L	23×13×7
Round Layer Cake Pan	8×1½	1.2 L	20×4
	9×1½	1.5 L	23×4
Pie Plate	8×1¼	750 mL	20×3
	9×1¼	1 L	23×3
Baking Dish or Casserole	1 quart	1 L	—
	1½ quart	1.5 L	—
	2 quart	2 L	—